D0515358

NURSING SCHUUL ENTRANCE EXAM FLASHCARDS

TEAS • NET • NLN PAX-RN • PSB-RN • C-NET-RN

TestWare® Edition

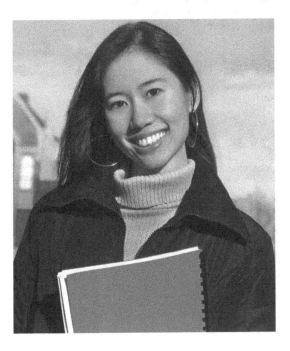

By The Staff of REA

Research & Education Association
Visit our website at: www.rea.com

Research & Education Association
61 Ethel Road West
Piscataway, New Jersey 08854
E-mail: info@rea.com

Nursing School Entrance Exam Flashcard Book with TestWare® on CD

Published 2016

Printed in the United States of America

ISBN-13: 978-0-7386-0894-5

ISBN-10: 0-7386-0894-7

About This Book

Being a Registered Nurse is an exciting, rewarding career, and REA wants you to succeed on your nursing school entrance exam so you can successfully enter a nursing program that will help you achieve your career goals. Wherever you take your test to enter a nursing program, you'll find this flashcard book to be perfect for self-study, for reference, or just for a quick review.

REA's unique flashcard book will help you succeed on various U.S. nursing school entrance exams, including the:

- **Test of Essential Academic Skills (TEAS)**
- **National League for Nursing Pre-Admission Examination (NLN PAX-RN)**
- **Nurse Entrance Test (NET)**
- **PSB Health Occupations Aptitude Exam**
- **C-NET Pre-Nursing Assessment Test-PN or -RN**

Nursing school entrance exams test the general knowledge needed for an education in nursing. To suit that need, the flashcards in this book are separated into different sections to match the format of various nursing school exams.

The **Mathematics/Numerical Ability** section will prepare you for items that test the following skills: conversion, decimals, distributive property, factoring, rate, unit price, fractions, negative numbers, operations, percentages, ratios, rounding, equations, square roots, price comparisons, digits, whole numbers, word problems, and writing expressions.

The **Verbal Ability** section will prepare you for items that test the following skills: analogies, antonyms, capitalization, language use, pronouns, punctuation, sentence structure, spelling, subject-verb agreement, and synonyms.

The **Science Ability** section will prepare you for items that test skills in biology, chemistry, and physics.

The **Reading Comprehension** section includes a short reading passage that will be referenced to answer several items that test skills in analysis, author's purpose, audience, cause and effect, drawing conclusions, evaluating information, main idea, inferences, sequencing, and text features.

In this TestWare® edition with CD-ROM, we've made it easy for you to hone your study skills. The accompanying CD offers you **four test-readiness quizzes** that will test how well you have absorbed the material. It's an excellent way to build knowledge and confidence.

Also included on the CD are four invaluable reference charts that you can return to time and again:

- **The Skeletal System;**

- **Circulatory System;**

- **Muscular System;** and

- **Anatomy and Physiology**

With this flashcard book, you won't have to deal with an awkward box and hundreds of loose cards. Here, everything you need to study is bound neatly inside, with questions on one side of a flashcard, a place to write your response, and the correct answer and a detailed explanation on the flip side of the card. It is portable and useful in many ways—for quick study, rapid review, and easy reference.

We are proud of this one-of-a-kind flashcard book, and we hope you find it valuable in your quest to launch your career in nursing.

Larry B. Kling
Chief Editor

Table of Contents

About Research & Education Association

Founded in 1959, Research & Education Association (REA) is dedicated to publishing the finest and most effective educational materials— including study guides and test preps—for students in middle school, high school, college, graduate school, and beyond.

Today, REA's wide-ranging catalog is a leading resource for teachers, students, and professionals. Visit *www.rea.com* to see a complete listing of all our titles.

Acknowledgments

We would like to thank Larry B. Kling, Vice President, Editorial, for his overall guidance, which brought this publication to completion; Pam Weston, Publisher, for setting the quality standards for production integrity and managing the publication to completion; John Cording, Vice President, Technology, for coordinating the design and development of REA's TestWare®; Diane Goldschmidt, Senior Editor, for project management; Alice Leonard and Kathleen Casey, Senior Editors, for preflight editorial review; Heena Patel, Technology Project Manager, for design contributions and software testing efforts; and Christine Saul, Senior Graphic Designer, for designing our cover.

We also gratefully acknowledge Words and Numbers for preparing the manuscript and DataStream Content Solutions for typesetting this edition.

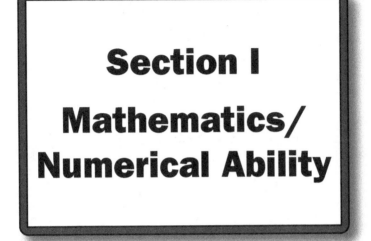

Section I

Mathematics/
Numerical Ability

Questions

Q–1

Which number shows three million, four hundred fifty-seven thousand, nine hundred forty?

(A) 345,794

(B) 3,457,940

(C) 34,579,040

(D) 300,457,940

Your Answer _____

Q–2

Round off 59,965 to the nearest hundred.

(A) 59,065

(B) 59,900

(C) 59,970

(D) 60,000

Your Answer _____

3

Correct Answers

A–1

(B) 3,457,940 is written as "three million, four hundred fifty-seven thousand, nine hundred forty." 345,794 is written as "three hundred forty-five thousand, seven hundred ninety-four." 34,579,040 is written as "thirty-four million, five hundred seventy-nine thousand, forty." 300,457,940 is written as "three hundred million, four hundred fifty-seven thousand, nine hundred forty."

A–2

(D) The "9" in the hundreds place is rounded up to 10. As a result, the "9" in the thousands place is rounded up to 10, which rounds the "5" in the ten thousands place up to 6. After all rounding is completed, 59,965 is rounded up to 60,000.

Questions

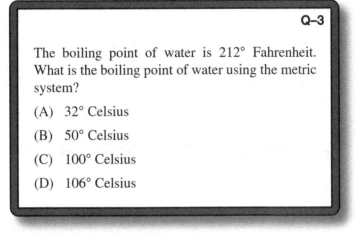

Q–3

The boiling point of water is 212° Fahrenheit. What is the boiling point of water using the metric system?

(A)   32° Celsius

(B)   50° Celsius

(C)   100° Celsius

(D)   106° Celsius

Your Answer ⎯⎯⎯⎯⎯⎯⎯⎯⎯⎯⎯⎯⎯⎯⎯⎯⎯⎯

⎯⎯⎯⎯⎯⎯⎯⎯⎯⎯⎯⎯⎯⎯⎯⎯⎯⎯⎯⎯⎯⎯⎯⎯⎯

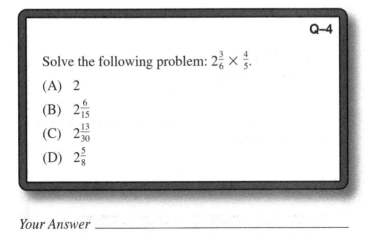

Q–4

Solve the following problem: $2\frac{3}{6} \times \frac{4}{5}$.

(A)   2

(B) $2\frac{6}{15}$

(C) $2\frac{13}{30}$

(D) $2\frac{5}{8}$

Your Answer ⎯⎯⎯⎯⎯⎯⎯⎯⎯⎯⎯⎯⎯⎯⎯⎯⎯⎯

⎯⎯⎯⎯⎯⎯⎯⎯⎯⎯⎯⎯⎯⎯⎯⎯⎯⎯⎯⎯⎯⎯⎯⎯

Correct Answers

A–3

(C)   In the metric system, 0° Celsius is the freezing point of water and 100° Celsius is the boiling point of water.

A–4

(A)   First, turn the mixed number $(2\frac{3}{6})$ into an improper fraction.

$$\frac{15}{6} \times \frac{4}{5}$$

Now, multiply the numerators together and the denominators together.

$$\frac{15}{6} \times \frac{4}{5} = \frac{60}{30}$$

$\frac{60}{30}$ can be reduced to 2.

Questions

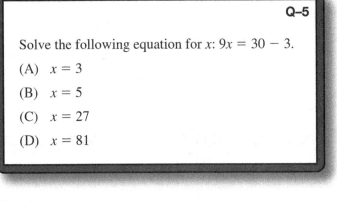

Q–5

Solve the following equation for x: $9x = 30 - 3$.

(A) $x = 3$

(B) $x = 5$

(C) $x = 27$

(D) $x = 81$

Your Answer _____

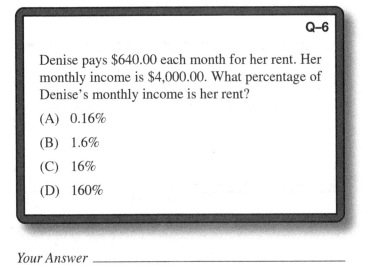

Q–6

Denise pays $640.00 each month for her rent. Her monthly income is $4,000.00. What percentage of Denise's monthly income is her rent?

(A) 0.16%

(B) 1.6%

(C) 16%

(D) 160%

Your Answer _____

Correct Answers

(A)   Simplify $9x = 30 - 3$.

$$9x = 27$$
$$x = 27 \div 9$$
$$x = 3$$

(C)   Denise's rent ($640.00) divided by her monthly salary ($4,000.00) is 0.16. 16% is equivalent to 0.16.

Questions

Q–7

Casper's Automotives produces 144 windshields in 8 hours. At what rate does Casper's Automotives produce windshields?

(A)   15 windshields per hour

(B)   16 windshields per hour

(C)   18 windshields per hour

(D)   20 windshields per hour

Your Answer _____

_____

Q–8

Solve the following problem: $(3 \times 3)^2 + 4(8 - 1)$.

(A)   37

(B)   59

(C)   109

(D)   595

Your Answer _____

_____

Correct Answers

A–7

(C)   To find the rate, divide the number of products made by the time it took to make them. The total number of windshields produced (144) divided by the time it took to produce the windshields (8 hours) yields a rate of 18 windshields per hour.

A–8

(C)   Follow the order of operations (PEMDAS). First, solve the problems in the parentheses.

$$(9)^2 + 4(7)$$

Then, work with the exponents.

$$81 + 4(7)$$

Next, solve the multiplication problem.

$$81 + 28$$

Finally, solve the addition problem.

$$81 + 28 = 109$$

Questions

Q–9

A patient has a temperature of 40.0° Celsius. What is the patient's temperature in degrees Fahrenheit?

(A) 97.0° Fahrenheit

(B) 98.6° Fahrenheit

(C) 100.2° Fahrenheit

(D) 104.0° Fahrenheit

Your Answer _____

_____

Q–10

Solve the following problem: $\frac{3}{4} \div \frac{7}{8}$.

(A) $\frac{3}{14}$

(B) $\frac{21}{32}$

(C) $\frac{6}{7}$

(D) $1\frac{1}{6}$

Your Answer _____

_____

Correct Answers

A–9

(D)   Use the following formula to convert from degrees Celsius to degrees Fahrenheit.

$$
\begin{aligned}
(\text{Degrees Celsius} \times 1.8) + 32 &= \text{Degrees Fahrenheit} \\
(40° \times 1.8) + 32 &= \text{Degrees Fahrenheit} \\
(72°) + 32 &= \text{Degrees Fahrenheit} \\
104° &= \text{Degrees Fahrenheit}
\end{aligned}
$$

A–10

(C)   First, "flip" $\frac{7}{8}$ to make it $\frac{8}{7}$.

$$\frac{3}{4} \div \frac{8}{7}$$

Instead of dividing, *multiply* the numerators with one another. Then, multiply the denominators with one another.

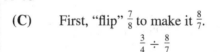

$$\frac{3}{4} \times \frac{8}{7} = \frac{24}{28}$$

$\frac{24}{28}$ can be reduced to $\frac{6}{7}$.

Questions

Q–11

Solve the following equation for x: $3x(3 + 6) = (9 \times 7) + 18x$.

(A) $x = 7$

(B) $x = 9$

(C) $x = 13$

(D) $x = 14$

Your Answer _____

Q–12

Mr. and Mrs. Harris pay $2,240.00 each month for their mortgage. Mr. Harris earns $2,600.00 each month. Mrs. Harris earns $3,000.00 each month. What percent of the Harrises' monthly income goes to pay the monthly mortgage?

(A) 3%

(B) 4%

(C) 30%

(D) 40%

Your Answer _____

Correct Answers

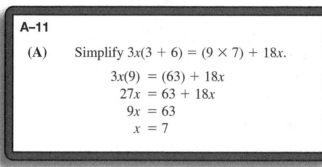

A–11

(A) Simplify $3x(3 + 6) = (9 \times 7) + 18x$.

$$3x(9) = (63) + 18x$$
$$27x = 63 + 18x$$
$$9x = 63$$
$$x = 7$$

A–12

(D) Add Mr. and Mrs. Harris's individual incomes to find their total monthly income.

$$\$2,600.00 + \$3,000.00 = \$5,600.00$$

Divide the monthly mortgage by the Harrises' monthly income.

$$\$2,240.00/\$5,600 = 0.4$$

40% is the equivalent of 0.4.

Questions

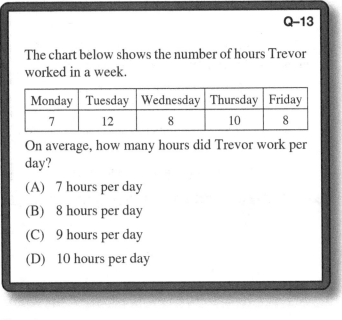

Q–13

The chart below shows the number of hours Trevor worked in a week.

Monday	Tuesday	Wednesday	Thursday	Friday
7	12	8	10	8

On average, how many hours did Trevor work per day?

(A)   7 hours per day

(B)   8 hours per day

(C)   9 hours per day

(D)   10 hours per day

Your Answer _____

_____

Correct Answers

A–13

(C) To find the find the average, calculate the number of hours Trevor worked in the week.

7 hours + 12 hours + 8 hours + 10 hours
$$+ \text{ 8 hours} = 45 \text{ hours}$$

Now divide the total number of hours (45) by the number of days worked.

45 hours/5 days = 9 hours per day

Questions

Q–14

David started a new job last year. The table shows his income by month.

First Half of the Year		Second Half of the Year	
Month	Monthly Income	Month	Monthly Income
January	$2,300.00	July	$2,700.00
February	$3,000.00	August	$3,100.00
March	$2,700.00	September	$2,900.00
April	$2,600.00	October	$2,200.00
May	$3,100.00	November	$2,800.00
June	$2,800.00	December	$3,000.00

Did David earn more money in the first half of the year or the second half of the year? By how much?

(A) He made $300.00 more in the first half of the year.

(B) He made $500.00 more in the first half of the year.

(C) He made $100.00 more in the second half of the year.

(D) He made $200.00 more in the second half of the year.

Your Answer _____

_____

Correct Answers

(D) First, add the months in each half of the year.

First Half of the Year	Second Half of the Year
$2,300.00	$2,700.00
$3,000.00	$3,100.00
$2,700.00	$2,900.00
$2,600.00	$2,200.00
$3,100.00	$2,800.00
+ $2,800.00	+ $3,000.00
$16,500.00	$16,700.00

David earned more money in the second half of the year. Now find the difference between the first half of the year and the second half of the year.

$$\begin{array}{r} \$16,700.00 \\ - \ \underline{\$16,500.00} \\ \$200.00 \end{array}$$

Questions

Q–15

There are 3.79 liters in a gallon. About how many liters are there in 12 gallons?

(A) 30 liters

(B) 35 liters

(C) 40 liters

(D) 45 liters

Your Answer _____

_____

Q–16

Solve the following problem: $\frac{10}{12} + \frac{8}{12}$.

(A) $1\frac{2}{12}$

(B) $1\frac{1}{2}$

(C) $1\frac{3}{4}$

(D) 2

Your Answer _____

_____

Correct Answers

A–15

(D) There are 3.79 liters in a gallon. 12 gallons multiplied by 3.79 liters per gallon is 45.48 liters. 45.48 rounds to 45.

A–16

(B) Because both fractions have a common denominator, simply add the numerators. The denominator will stay the same.

$$\frac{10}{12} + \frac{8}{12} = \frac{18}{12}$$

$\frac{18}{12}$ is an improper fraction that is equivalent to $1\frac{6}{12}$. Next, reduce $1\frac{6}{12}$ to $1\frac{1}{2}$.

Questions

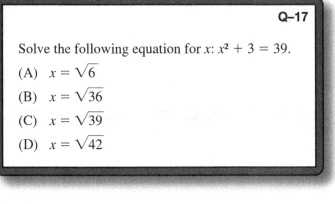

Q–17

Solve the following equation for x: $x^2 + 3 = 39$.

(A) $x = \sqrt{6}$

(B) $x = \sqrt{36}$

(C) $x = \sqrt{39}$

(D) $x = \sqrt{42}$

Your Answer _____

_____

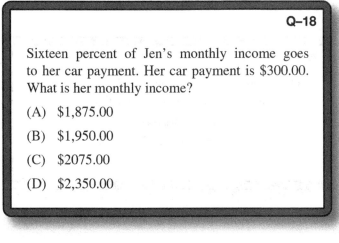

Q–18

Sixteen percent of Jen's monthly income goes to her car payment. Her car payment is $300.00. What is her monthly income?

(A) $1,875.00

(B) $1,950.00

(C) $2075.00

(D) $2,350.00

Your Answer _____

_____

Correct Answers

A–17

(B)   Simplify $x^2 - 3 = 39$.

$$x^2 = 36$$
$$x = \sqrt{36}$$

A–18

(A)   Set up an equation to solve the problem. 0.16 is the decimal equivalent of 16%.

$$0.16x = \$300.00$$
$$x = \$300.00 \div 0.16$$
$$x = \$1,875.00$$

Questions

Q–19

Molly drove six hours at an average rate of 55 miles per hour. How far did Molly travel?

(A) 315 miles

(B) 330 miles

(C) 345 miles

(D) 360 miles

Your Answer _____

_____

Q–20

Solve the following problem: $1,458 - 378 + 3,066$.

(A) 4,038

(B) 4,146

(C) 4,350

(D) 4,902

Your Answer _____

_____

Correct Answers

A–19

(B)   To find the distance traveled, multiply the time (6 hours) by the rate (55 miles per hour).

6 hours × 55 miles per hour = 330 miles

A–20

(B)   First, solve the subtraction problem.

$$1,458 - 378 = 1,080$$

Then, add 3,066 to the difference.

$$1,080 + 3,066 = 4,146$$

Questions

Q–21

There are about 0.6 miles in one kilometer. If Megan travels 240 miles, about how far has she traveled in kilometers?

(A) 350 kilometers

(B) 400 kilometers

(C) 450 kilometers

(D) 500 kilometers

Your Answer _____

_____

Q–22

Jackie is taking two courses this semester. Her anatomy class is three credits and costs $295.50 per credit. Her biology class is four credits and costs $270.10 per credit. How much will Jackie pay in tuition this semester?

(A) $1,080.40

(B) $1,696.80

(C) $1,890.50

(D) $1,966.90

Your Answer _____

_____

Correct Answers

A–21

(B) There are about 0.6 miles in a kilometer. 240 miles divided by 0.6 miles in a kilometer is 400 kilometers.

A–22

(D) First, find the cost of each class.

Anatomy: 3 credits × $295.50 = $886.50
Biology: 4 credits × $270.10 = $1,080.40

Then, add the total costs of the classes.

$886.50 + $1,080.40 = $1,966.90

Questions

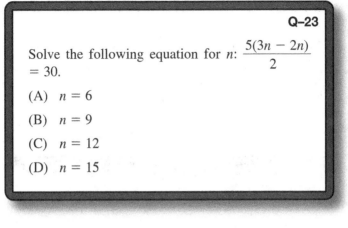

Q–23

Solve the following equation for n: $\dfrac{5(3n - 2n)}{2} = 30$.

(A) $n = 6$

(B) $n = 9$

(C) $n = 12$

(D) $n = 15$

Your Answer _____

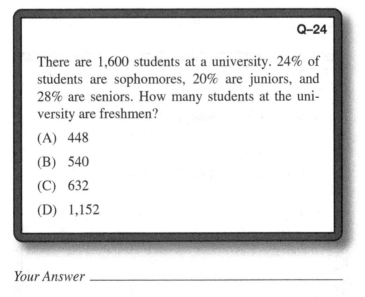

Q–24

There are 1,600 students at a university. 24% of students are sophomores, 20% are juniors, and 28% are seniors. How many students at the university are freshmen?

(A) 448

(B) 540

(C) 632

(D) 1,152

Your Answer _____

Correct Answers

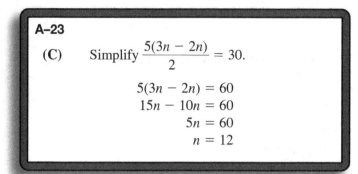

A–23

(C) Simplify $\dfrac{5(3n - 2n)}{2} = 30$.

$$5(3n - 2n) = 60$$
$$15n - 10n = 60$$
$$5n = 60$$
$$n = 12$$

A–24

(A) In order to find the percentage of students who are freshmen, subtract the percentages of sophomores (24%), juniors (20%), and seniors (28%) from 100%.

$$100\% - (24\% + 20\% + 28\%) = ?$$
$$100\% - (72\%) = 28\% \text{ freshmen}$$

Now multiply the percentage of students that are freshmen (28%) by the student population of the university (1,600). 0.28 is equivalent to 28%.

$$0.28 \times 1,600 = 448$$

Questions

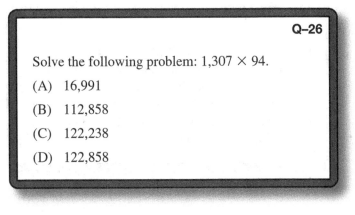

Q–25

NiteTime Cough Relief comes in four bottle sizes: 12 ounces, 15 ounces, 18 ounces, and 24 ounces. Four people purchased NiteTime Cough Relief. Who got the best price?

	Amanda	Becca	Chris	D'Arcy
Size	15 ounces	12 ounces	24 ounces	18 ounces
Price	$9.75	$9.00	$16.32	$12.96

(A) Amanda

(B) Becca

(C) Chris

(D) D'Arcy

Your Answer _____

Q–26

Solve the following problem: 1,307 × 94.

(A) 16,991

(B) 112,858

(C) 122,238

(D) 122,858

Your Answer _____

29

Correct Answers

A–25

(A) The total cost of Amanda's bottle ($9.75) divided by the amount (15 ounces) yields a unit price of $0.65. The total cost of Becca's bottle ($9.00) divided by the amount (12 ounces) yields a unit price of $0.75. The total cost of Chris's bottle ($16.32) divided by the amount (24 ounces) yields a unit price of $0.68. The total cost of D'Arcy's bottle ($12.96) divided by the amount (18 ounces) yields a unit price of $0.72.

A–26

(D) The product of 1,307 and 94 is 122,858. An answer of 16,991 indicates that a "0" placeholder was not used in the ones column. An answer of 112,858 neglects to carry the "1" from the thousands column. An answer of 122,238 indicates two multiplication errors.

Questions

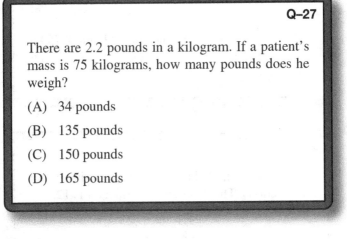

Q–27

There are 2.2 pounds in a kilogram. If a patient's mass is 75 kilograms, how many pounds does he weigh?

(A) 34 pounds

(B) 135 pounds

(C) 150 pounds

(D) 165 pounds

Your Answer _____

_____

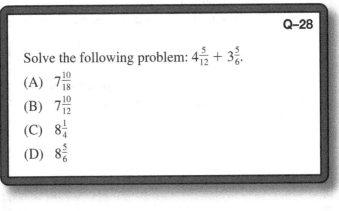

Q–28

Solve the following problem: $4\frac{5}{12} + 3\frac{5}{6}$.

(A) $7\frac{10}{18}$

(B) $7\frac{10}{12}$

(C) $8\frac{1}{4}$

(D) $8\frac{5}{6}$

Your Answer _____

_____

Correct Answers

A–27

(D) There are 2.2 pounds in a kilogram. 75 kilograms multiplied by 2.2 pounds in a kilogram is 165 pounds.

A–28

(C) First, find the common denominator for the fractions. The common denominator is 12.

$$4\tfrac{5}{12} \qquad 4\tfrac{5}{12}$$
$$+\ 3\tfrac{5}{6} = +\ 3\tfrac{?}{12}$$

Now, find the numerator that will make $\tfrac{5}{6}$ equivalent to $\tfrac{?}{12}$. The new numerator is 10 because $\tfrac{5}{6}$ is equivalent to $\tfrac{10}{12}$.

$$4\tfrac{5}{12} \qquad 4\tfrac{5}{12}$$
$$+\ 3\tfrac{5}{6} = +\ 3\tfrac{10}{12}$$

Add the fractions: $\tfrac{5}{12} + \tfrac{10}{12} = \tfrac{15}{12}$. This is an improper fraction (meaning a fraction that is larger than 1) because the numerator is larger than the denominator. Turn $\tfrac{15}{12}$ into a mixed number and the result is $1\tfrac{3}{12}$.

$$\tfrac{15}{12} = 1\tfrac{3}{12}$$

The 1 from the mixed number can be added to the other two whole numbers in the problem: $4 + 3 + 1 = 8$.

$$
\begin{aligned}
4 \\
3 \\
+\ 1\tfrac{3}{12} \\
\hline
8\tfrac{3}{12}
\end{aligned}
$$

Finally, $8\tfrac{3}{12}$ can be reduced to $8\tfrac{1}{4}$.

Questions

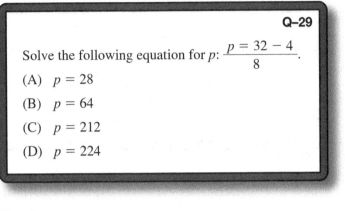

Q-29

Solve the following equation for p: $\dfrac{p = 32 - 4}{8}$.

(A) $p = 28$

(B) $p = 64$

(C) $p = 212$

(D) $p = 224$

Your Answer _____

_____

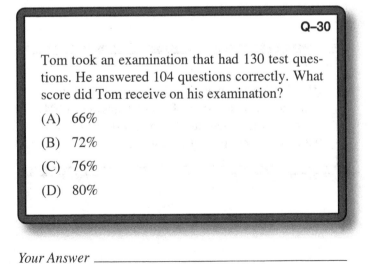

Q-30

Tom took an examination that had 130 test questions. He answered 104 questions correctly. What score did Tom receive on his examination?

(A) 66%

(B) 72%

(C) 76%

(D) 80%

Your Answer _____

_____

Correct Answers

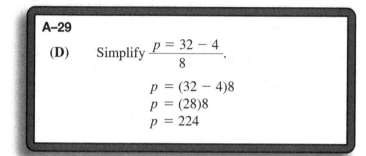

A–29

(D)   Simplify $\dfrac{p = 32 - 4}{8}$.

$$p = (32 - 4)8$$
$$p = (28)8$$
$$p = 224$$

A–30

(D)   Tom answered 104 out of 130 questions correctly. The number of correct answers (104) divided by the total number of questions (130) is 0.80. 80% is equivalent to 0.80.

Questions

Q–31

A grocery store sells cans of four types of soup in various sizes.

	MacAllen's Soup	Farmer's Soup	Sun Valley Soup	Just Like Home Soup
Size	24 ounces	20 ounces	16 ounces	28 ounces
Price	$2.88	$2.60	$2.24	$3.08

Which soup has the lowest price per ounce?

(A) MacAllen's Soup

(B) Farmer's Soup

(C) Sun Valley Soup

(D) Just Like Home Soup

Your Answer ⎯⎯⎯⎯⎯⎯⎯⎯⎯⎯⎯⎯⎯⎯⎯⎯

⎯⎯⎯⎯⎯⎯⎯⎯⎯⎯⎯⎯⎯⎯⎯⎯⎯⎯⎯⎯⎯⎯⎯⎯

Correct Answers

A–31

(D)   The total cost of Just Like Home Soup ($3.08) divided by the amount (28 ounces) yields a unit price of $0.11. The total cost of MacAllen's Soup ($2.88) divided by the amount (24 ounces) yields a unit price of $0.12. The total cost of Farmer's Soup ($2.60) divided by the amount (20 ounces) yields a unit price of $0.13. The total cost of Sun Valley Soup ($2.24) divided by the amount (16 ounces) yields a unit price of $0.14.

Questions

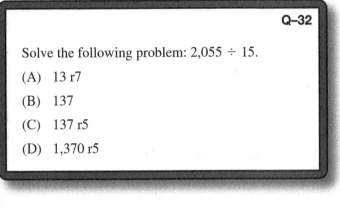

Q–32

Solve the following problem: 2,055 ÷ 15.

(A) 13 r7

(B) 137

(C) 137 r5

(D) 1,370 r5

Your Answer _____

_____

Correct Answers

(B)   The quotient of 2,005 ÷ 15 is 137.

First, find how many times 15 can go into 20. It can go in one time.

$$\overset{1}{15\overline{)2,055}}$$

Then, multiply 1 by 15. Subtract that from 20.

$$
\begin{array}{r}
1 \\
15\overline{)2,055} \\
-15 \\
\hline
5
\end{array}
$$

Next, bring down the 5 from the tens column. You now have 55.

$$
\begin{array}{r}
1 \\
15\overline{)2,055} \\
-15 \\
\hline
55
\end{array}
$$

How many times can 15 go into 55? It can go in three times.

$$
\begin{array}{r}
13 \\
15\overline{)2,055} \\
-15 \\
\hline
55
\end{array}
$$

Next, multiply 3 by 15. Subtract that from 55.

$$
\begin{array}{r}
13 \\
15\overline{)2,055} \\
-15 \\
\hline
55 \\
-45 \\
\hline
10
\end{array}
$$

(Continued)

Correct Answers

Now bring down the 5 from the ones column. You now have 105.

$$
\begin{array}{r}
13 \\
15\,)\,\overline{2{,}055} \\
-\,15 \\
\hline
55 \\
-\,45 \\
\hline
105
\end{array}
$$

How many times can 15 go into 105? It can go in seven times.

$$
\begin{array}{r}
137 \\
15\,)\,\overline{2{,}055} \\
-\,15 \\
\hline
55 \\
-\,45 \\
\hline
105
\end{array}
$$

Next, multiply 7 by 15. Subtract that from 105.

$$
\begin{array}{r}
137 \\
15\,)\,\overline{2{,}055} \\
-\,15 \\
\hline
55 \\
-\,45 \\
\hline
105 \\
-\,105 \\
\hline
0
\end{array}
$$

Questions

Q–33

There are 2.2 pounds in a kilogram. If a patient weighs 198 pounds, what is his mass in kilograms?

(A)   86 kilograms

(B)   90 kilograms

(C)   430 kilograms

(D)   436 kilograms

Your Answer _____

_____

Correct Answers

A–33

(B)   There are 2.2 pounds in a kilogram. 198 pounds divided by 2.2 pounds in a kilogram is 90 kilograms.

Questions

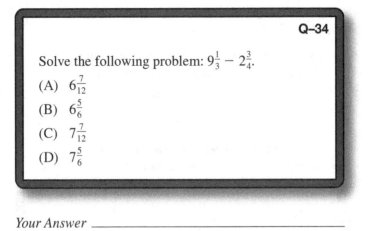

Q–34

Solve the following problem: $9\frac{1}{3} - 2\frac{3}{4}$.

(A) $6\frac{7}{12}$

(B) $6\frac{5}{6}$

(C) $7\frac{7}{12}$

(D) $7\frac{5}{6}$

Your Answer _____

_____

Correct Answers

A–34

(A) First, find the common denominator for the fractions. The common denominator is 12.

$$9\tfrac{1}{3} \qquad 9\tfrac{?}{12}$$
$$-2\tfrac{3}{4} = -2\tfrac{?}{12}$$

Now find the numerator that will make $\tfrac{1}{3}$ equivalent to $\tfrac{?}{12}$. The new numerator is 4 because $\tfrac{1}{3}$ is equivalent to $\tfrac{4}{12}$.

$$9\tfrac{1}{3} \qquad 9\tfrac{4}{12}$$
$$-2\tfrac{3}{4} = -2\tfrac{?}{12}$$

Next, find the numerator that will make $\tfrac{3}{4}$ equivalent to $\tfrac{?}{12}$. The new numerator is 9 because $\tfrac{3}{4}$ is equivalent to $\tfrac{9}{12}$.

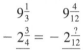

$$9\tfrac{1}{3} \qquad 9\tfrac{4}{12}$$
$$-2\tfrac{3}{4} = -2\tfrac{9}{12}$$

The next step is to subtract the fractions. However, $\tfrac{4}{12}$ is less than $\tfrac{9}{12}$. In order to make subtracting the fractions possible, $\tfrac{4}{12}$ must borrow 1 from the whole number 9. Add the denominator to the numerator. The 9 becomes an 8 because the fraction borrowed 1.

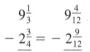

$$8\tfrac{16}{12}$$
$$-2\tfrac{9}{12}$$

Now subtract the whole numbers and the fractions.

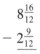

$$8\tfrac{16}{12}$$
$$-2\tfrac{9}{12} = 6\tfrac{7}{12}$$

$6\tfrac{7}{12}$ cannot be reduced.

Questions

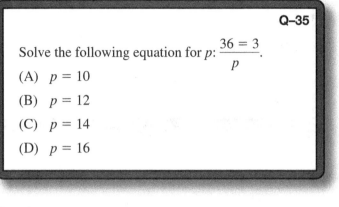

Q–35

Solve the following equation for p: $\dfrac{36 = 3}{p}$.

(A) $p = 10$

(B) $p = 12$

(C) $p = 14$

(D) $p = 16$

Your Answer _____

_____

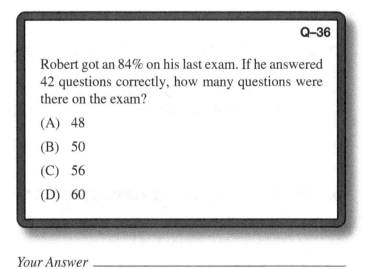

Q–36

Robert got an 84% on his last exam. If he answered 42 questions correctly, how many questions were there on the exam?

(A) 48

(B) 50

(C) 56

(D) 60

Your Answer _____

_____

Correct Answers

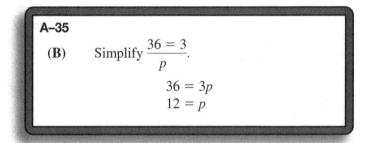

A–35

(B)   Simplify $\dfrac{36 = 3}{p}$.

$$36 = 3p$$
$$12 = p$$

A–36

(B)   Set up an equation to solve the problem. 0.84 is the decimal equivalent of 84%.

$$0.84x = 42$$
$$x = 42 \div 0.84$$
$$x = 50$$

Questions

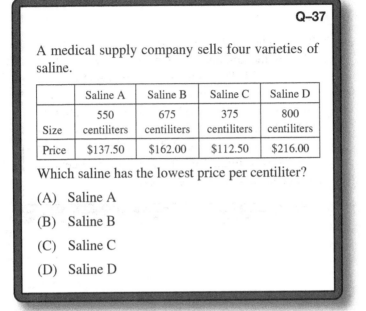

Q–37

A medical supply company sells four varieties of saline.

	Saline A	Saline B	Saline C	Saline D
Size	550 centiliters	675 centiliters	375 centiliters	800 centiliters
Price	$137.50	$162.00	$112.50	$216.00

Which saline has the lowest price per centiliter?

(A) Saline A

(B) Saline B

(C) Saline C

(D) Saline D

Your Answer _____

Q–38

Carmen took four exams this semester. Her scores were 80%, 78%, 84%, and 98%. What was Carmen's average score for the semester?

(A) 80%

(B) 83%

(C) 85%

(D) 88%

Your Answer _____

Correct Answers

A–37

(B) The total cost of Saline B ($162.00) divided by the amount (675 centiliters) yields a unit price of $0.24. The total cost of Saline A ($137.50) divided by the amount (550 centiliters) yields a unit price of $0.25. The total cost of Saline C ($112.50) divided by the amount (375 centiliters) yields a unit price of $0.30. The total cost of Saline D ($200.00) divided by the amount (800 centiliters) yields a unit price of $0.27.

A–38

(C) To find an average score, first add all the scores together.

$$80 + 78 + 84 + 98 = 340$$

Then, divide the total score (340) by the number of exams (4).

$$340 \div 4 = 85$$

Questions

Q–39

If it is 86° Fahrenheit outside, what is the temperature in degrees Celsius?

(A) 28° Celsius

(B) 30° Celsius

(C) 32° Celsius

(D) 35° Celsius

Your Answer _____

_____

Q–40

What is $\frac{5}{6}$ of 8?

(A) 6

(B) $6\frac{1}{4}$

(C) $6\frac{3}{8}$

(D) $6\frac{2}{3}$

Your Answer _____

_____

Correct Answers

A–39

(B) Use the following formula to convert from degrees Celsius to degrees Fahrenheit.

$$\frac{(\text{Degrees Fahrenheit} - 32)}{9} \times 5 = \text{Degrees Celsius}$$

$$\frac{(86° - 32)}{9} \times 5 = \text{Degrees Celsius}$$

$$\frac{(54) \times 5}{9} = \text{Degrees Celsius}$$

$$\frac{270}{9} = \text{Degrees Celsius}$$

$$30° = \text{Degrees Celsius}$$

A–40

(D) First, turn 8 into a fraction by placing a 1 in the denominator.

$$\frac{5}{6} \times \frac{8}{1}$$

Now multiply the numerators. Then, multiply the denominators.

$$\frac{5}{6} \times \frac{8}{1} = \frac{40}{6}$$

$\frac{40}{6}$ is equivalent to $6\frac{4}{6}$.

$6\frac{4}{6}$ can be reduced to $6\frac{2}{3}$.

Questions

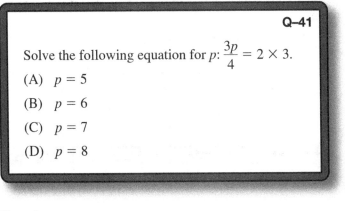

Q–41

Solve the following equation for p: $\dfrac{3p}{4} = 2 \times 3$.

(A) $p = 5$

(B) $p = 6$

(C) $p = 7$

(D) $p = 8$

Your Answer _____

_____

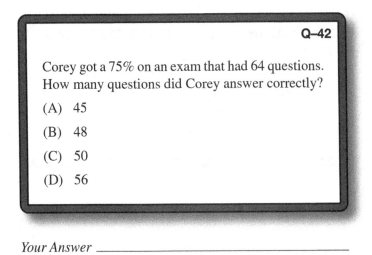

Q–42

Corey got a 75% on an exam that had 64 questions. How many questions did Corey answer correctly?

(A) 45

(B) 48

(C) 50

(D) 56

Your Answer _____

_____

Correct Answers

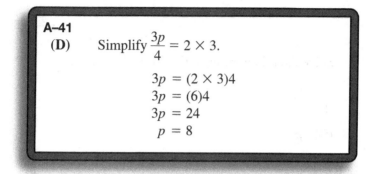

A–41

(D)   Simplify $\dfrac{3p}{4} = 2 \times 3.$

$$3p = (2 \times 3)4$$
$$3p = (6)4$$
$$3p = 24$$
$$p = 8$$

A–42

(B)   0.75 is equivalent to 75%. Multiply the total number of questions (64) by the percentage of questions answered correctly (0.75).

$$64 \times 0.75 = 48$$

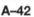

Questions

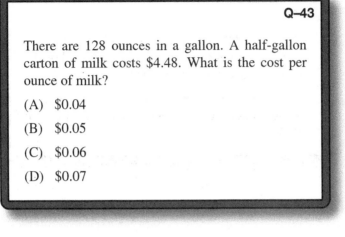

Q–43

There are 128 ounces in a gallon. A half-gallon carton of milk costs $4.48. What is the cost per ounce of milk?

(A) $0.04

(B) $0.05

(C) $0.06

(D) $0.07

Your Answer _____

_____

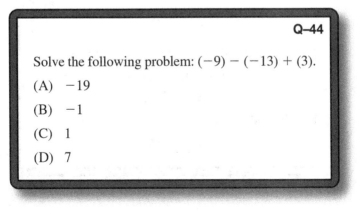

Q–44

Solve the following problem: $(-9) - (-13) + (3)$.

(A) -19

(B) -1

(C) 1

(D) 7

Your Answer _____

_____

Correct Answers

A–43

(D)   Find the number of ounces in a half gallon of milk. One gallon (128 ounces) multiplied by the percent of one gallon (50%) is 64 ounces.

The total cost of the carton of milk ($4.48) divided by the amount (64 ounces) yields a unit price of $0.07.

A–44

(D)   First, solve the subtraction problem.

$(-9) - (-13)$ is the same as $(-9) + 13$.
$$-9 + 13 = 4$$

Finally, add 3 to the sum.

$$4 + 3 = 7$$

Questions

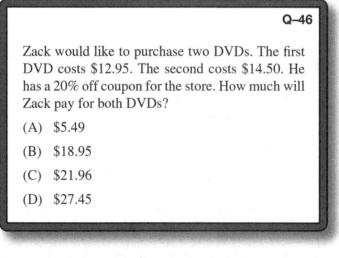

Q–45

There are 454 grams in a pound. If a patient weighs 132 pounds, what is her mass in kilograms?

(A)   5.8 kilograms

(B)   6.0 kilograms

(C)   58.0 kilograms

(D)   60.0 kilograms

Your Answer _____

_____

Q–46

Zack would like to purchase two DVDs. The first DVD costs $12.95. The second costs $14.50. He has a 20% off coupon for the store. How much will Zack pay for both DVDs?

(A) $5.49

(B) $18.95

(C) $21.96

(D) $27.45

Your Answer _____

_____

Correct Answers

A–45

(D) There are 454 grams in a pound. There are 1,000 grams in a kilogram. 454 grams in a pound divided by 1,000 grams in a kilogram is 0.454 kilograms in a pound.

Now multiply the patient's weight (132 pounds) by the number of kilograms in a pound (0.454).

132 pounds × 0.454 kilograms in a pound is 59.928 kilograms.

59.928 rounds to 60.0.

A–46

(C) First, add the costs of the two DVDs.

$$\$12.95 + \$14.50 = \$27.45$$

Now find 20% of the total. 0.20 is equivalent to 20%.

$$\$27.45 \times 0.20 = \$5.49$$

Finally, subtract the discount from the total price.

$$\$27.45 - \$5.49 = \$21.96$$

Questions

Q-47

Solve the following equation for n: $n = \dfrac{64}{n}$.

(A) $n = 8, -8$

(B) $n = 16, -16$

(C) $n = 24, -24$

(D) $n = 32, -32$

Your Answer _____

Q-48

John has a monthly income of $3,820.00. His monthly mortgage is $1,375.20. What percentage of John's monthly income remains after he pays his mortgage?

(A) 36%

(B) 48%

(C) 58%

(D) 64%

Your Answer _____

Correct Answers

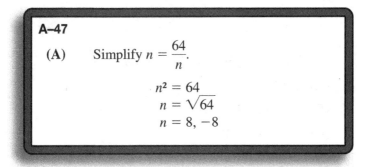

(A)   Simplify $n = \dfrac{64}{n}$.

$$n^2 = 64$$
$$n = \sqrt{64}$$
$$n = 8, -8$$

A–48

(D)   First, find the percentage of income that goes to rent. Divide the rent ($1,375.20) by John's monthly income ($3,820.00).

$$\$1,375.20 \div \$3,820.00 = 0.36$$

36% is equivalent to 0.36.

Now subtract the percentage of income that goes to rent (36%) from 100% to find what percentage of John's income remains.

$$100\% - 36\% = 64\%$$

Questions

Q–49

Theresa read 144 pages of her textbook in four and a half hours. At what rate did Theresa read?

(A) 32 pages per hour

(B) 35 pages per hour

(C) 36 pages per hour

(D) 38 pages per hour

Your Answer _____

_____

Q–50

Solve the following problem: 4,517 + 923 + 12,409.

(A) 16,849

(B) 17,839

(C) 17,849

(D) 26,156

Your Answer _____

_____

Correct Answers

A–49

(A)   Divide the number of pages (144) by the length of time it took to read those pages (4.5 hours).

$$144 \div 4.5 = 32$$

A–50

(C)   The sum of 4,517, 923, and 12,409 is 17,849. An answer of 16,849 neglects to carry the "1" from the hundreds column. An answer of 17,839 neglects to carry the "1" from the ones column. An answer of 26,156 indicates that 923 was not properly aligned.

Questions

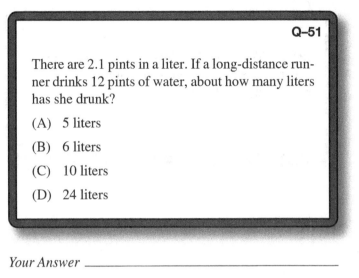

Q–51

There are 2.1 pints in a liter. If a long-distance runner drinks 12 pints of water, about how many liters has she drunk?

(A)   5 liters

(B)   6 liters

(C)   10 liters

(D)   24 liters

Your Answer _____

_____

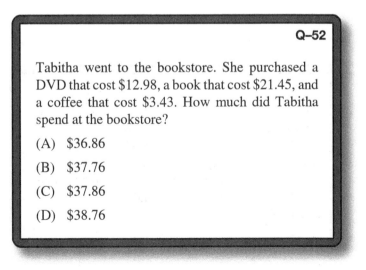

Q–52

Tabitha went to the bookstore. She purchased a DVD that cost $12.98, a book that cost $21.45, and a coffee that cost $3.43. How much did Tabitha spend at the bookstore?

(A) $36.86

(B) $37.76

(C) $37.86

(D) $38.76

Your Answer _____

_____

Correct Answers

A–51

(B) There are 2.1 pints in a liter. 12 pints of water divided by 2.1 pints in a liter is 5.7. 5.7 is rounded up to 6 liters.

A–52

(C) Tabitha's purchases totaled $37.86. An answer of $36.86 neglects to carry the "1" in the tenths column. An answer of $37.76 neglects to carry the "1" in the hundredths column. An answer of $38.76 carries the "1's" from both the hundredths and tenths columns and adds them to the ones column.

Questions

Q–53

Factor the following expression: $x^2 - 5x - 36$.

(A) $(x - 5)(x - 36)$

(B) $(x - 5x)(x - 36)$

(C) $(x + 4)(x - 9)$

(D) $(x + 9)(x - 4)$

Your Answer _____

_____

Q–54

Cheryl has $4,400.00 in her savings account. Her savings account earned her 6% in interest. How much interest did Cheryl gain?

(A) $264.00

(B) $270.00

(C) $284.00

(D) $290.00

Your Answer _____

_____

Correct Answers

A–53

(C)   The first term in both sets of parentheses must be x in order to have x^2.

$$(x \pm \_)(x \pm \_)$$

The second terms in both sets of parentheses must have a sum of -5 and a product of -36. So the second terms must be 4 and -9.

$$(x + 4)(x - 9)$$

A–54

(A)   0.06 is the decimal equivalent of 6%. $4,400.00 multiplied by 0.06 is $264.00.

Questions

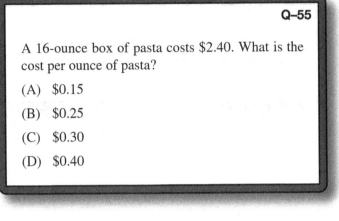

Q-55

A 16-ounce box of pasta costs $2.40. What is the cost per ounce of pasta?

(A) $0.15

(B) $0.25

(C) $0.30

(D) $0.40

Your Answer _____

_____

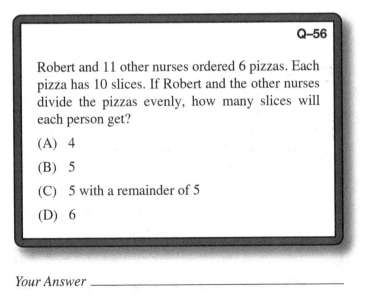

Q-56

Robert and 11 other nurses ordered 6 pizzas. Each pizza has 10 slices. If Robert and the other nurses divide the pizzas evenly, how many slices will each person get?

(A) 4

(B) 5

(C) 5 with a remainder of 5

(D) 6

Your Answer _____

_____

Correct Answers

A–55

(A)   The total cost of the box of pasta ($2.40) divided by the amount (16 ounces) yields a unit price of $0.15.

A–56

(B)   There are a total of 12 people ordering pizza, including Robert. To find the total number of slices, multiply the number of pizzas (6) by the number of slices in each pizza (10).

$$6 \times 10 = 60$$

Now divide the total number of slices (60) by the number of people who ordered pizza (12).

$$60 \div 12 = 5$$

Questions

Q–57

There are 3.79 liters in a gallon. If a hospital orders 150 gallons of saline, about how much saline has the hospital ordered in liters?

(A) 39 liters

(B) 40 liters

(C) 560 liters

(D) 570 liters

Your Answer _____

_____

Q–58

Twelve nursing students go to dinner. The bill of $341.76 includes tip. If the students split the bill evenly, how much money does each student owe?

(A) $26.40

(B) $28.48

(C) $30.36

(D) $34.17

Your Answer _____

_____

Correct Answers

A–57

(D) There are 3.79 liters in a gallon. 150 gallons multiplied by 3.79 liters in a gallon is 568.5 liters. 568.5 liters is rounded up to 570 liters.

A–58

(B) To solve the problem, divide the total bill ($341.76) by the number of students (12). The quotient is $28.48.

Questions

Q–59

Solve the following equation for x: $6(x + 4) = (1 + x)9$.

(A) 4

(B) 5

(C) 6

(D) 7

Your Answer _____

_____

Q–60

David wants to buy a new car that costs $15,280.00. However, this price does not include taxes. The taxes are 8% of the cost of the car. How much will David pay for the car?

(A) $15,678.76

(B) $15,890.60

(C) $16,436.84

(D) $16,502.40

Your Answer _____

_____

Correct Answers

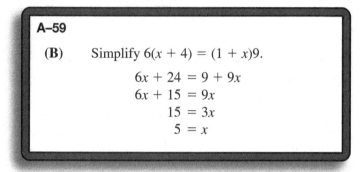

A–59

(B)   Simplify $6(x + 4) = (1 + x)9$.

$$6x + 24 = 9 + 9x$$
$$6x + 15 = 9x$$
$$15 = 3x$$
$$5 = x$$

A–60

(D)   0.08 is the decimal equivalent of 8%. $15,280 multiplied by 0.08 is $1,222.40. The tax on the car is $1,222.40. Add the tax ($1,222.40) to the price of the car ($15,280.00), and the total cost is $16,502.40.

Questions

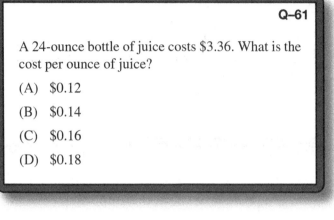

Q–61

A 24-ounce bottle of juice costs $3.36. What is the cost per ounce of juice?

(A) $0.12

(B) $0.14

(C) $0.16

(D) $0.18

Your Answer _____

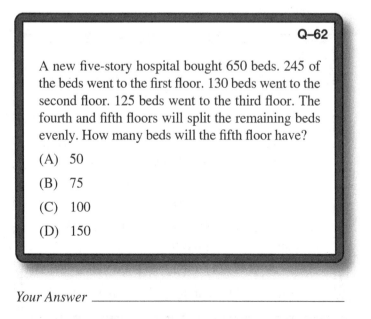

Q–62

A new five-story hospital bought 650 beds. 245 of the beds went to the first floor. 130 beds went to the second floor. 125 beds went to the third floor. The fourth and fifth floors will split the remaining beds evenly. How many beds will the fifth floor have?

(A) 50

(B) 75

(C) 100

(D) 150

Your Answer _____

Correct Answers

A-61

(B) The total cost of the bottle of juice ($3.36) divided by the amount (24 ounces) yields a unit price of $0.14.

A-62

(B) First, add the number of beds being sent to the first, second, and third floors.

$$245 + 130 + 125 = 500$$

Next, subtract the number of beds going to the first, second, and third floors (500) from the total number of beds (650).

$$650 - 500 = 150$$

Now divide the number of beds left over (150) by the number of floors left over (2).

$$150 \div 2 = 75$$

The fourth and fifth floors will each have 75 beds.

Questions

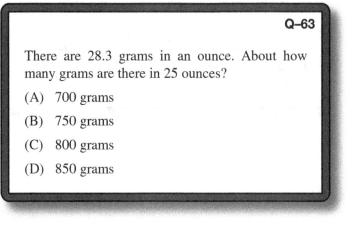

Q–63

There are 28.3 grams in an ounce. About how many grams are there in 25 ounces?

(A) 700 grams

(B) 750 grams

(C) 800 grams

(D) 850 grams

Your Answer _____

_____

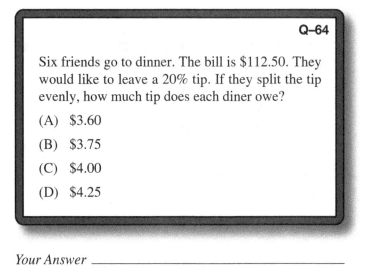

Q–64

Six friends go to dinner. The bill is $112.50. They would like to leave a 20% tip. If they split the tip evenly, how much tip does each diner owe?

(A) $3.60

(B) $3.75

(C) $4.00

(D) $4.25

Your Answer _____

_____

Correct Answers

A–63

(A) There are 28.3 grams in an ounce. 25 ounces multiplied by 28.3 grams per ounce is 707.5 grams. 707.5 rounds to 700.

A–64

(B) First, find out how much 20% of $112.50 is. Turn the 20% into a decimal and multiply.

$$\$112.50 \times 0.20 = \$22.50$$

Then, divide the tip ($22.50) by the number of diners.

$$\$22.50 \div 6 = \$3.75$$

Questions

Q–65

Solve the following equation for n: $5.8n + 12 = 99$.

(A) $n = 14.12$

(B) $n = 15$

(C) $n = 17.4$

(D) $n = 18$

Your Answer _____

_____

Correct Answers

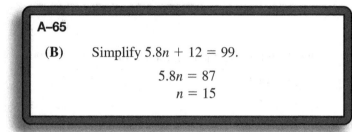

A–65

(B) Simplify $5.8n + 12 = 99$.

$$5.8n = 87$$
$$n = 15$$

Questions

Q-66

This is Anna's monthly budget.

Item	Income	Expense
Office Salary	$2,500	
Tutoring Income	$350.00	
Rent		$750.00
Car Payment		$350.00
Tuition		$570.00
Credit Card Bill		$220.00

What percentage of Anna's total monthly income goes to tuition?

(A) 16.5%

(B) 18.0%

(C) 19.0%

(D) 20.0%

Your Answer _____

Correct Answers

A–66

(D) First, find Anna's total monthly income by adding her office salary ($2,500.00) to her tutoring income ($350.00).

$$\$2,500.00 + \$350.00 = \$2,850.00$$

Then divide her tuition ($570.00) by her total monthly income ($2,850.00).

$$\$570.00 \div \$2,850.00 = 0.2.$$

20% is equivalent to 0.2.

Questions

The ratio of people in an audience is 5:2 females to males. If there are 80 females in the audience, how many total people are in the audience?

(A)   106

(B)   112

(C)   118

(D)   124

Your Answer _____

_____

Solve the following problem: $\dfrac{(3 + 9)}{2} + (3 \times 7)^2$.

(A)   406

(B)   435

(C)   447

(D)   453

Your Answer _____

_____

Correct Answers

A–67

(B) Set up a ratio to find the number of males in the audience.

$$\frac{5}{2} = \frac{80 \text{ females}}{x \text{ males}}$$

Now, cross multiply.

$$(2)(80 \text{ females}) = (5)(x \text{ males})$$
$$160 = 5x$$
$$32 \text{ males} = x$$

Now add the number of females (80) to the number of males (32).

$$80 + 32 = 112$$

A–68

(C) Follow the order of operations (PEMDAS). First, solve the problems in the parentheses.

$$\frac{(12)}{2} + (21)^2$$

Then, work with the exponent.

$$\frac{(12)}{2} + 441$$

Now solve the division problem.

$$6 + 441$$

Finally, solve the addition problem.

$$6 + 441 = 447$$

Questions

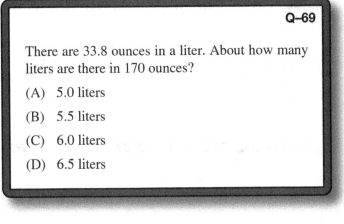

Q-69

There are 33.8 ounces in a liter. About how many liters are there in 170 ounces?

(A)   5.0 liters

(B)   5.5 liters

(C)   6.0 liters

(D)   6.5 liters

Your Answer _____

Correct Answers

A–69

(A)   There are 33.8 ounces in a liter. 170 ounces divided by 33.8 ounces in a liter is 5.03 liters. 5.03 rounds to 5.0.

Questions

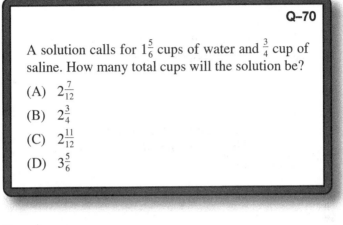

Q–70

A solution calls for $1\frac{5}{6}$ cups of water and $\frac{3}{4}$ cup of saline. How many total cups will the solution be?

(A) $2\frac{7}{12}$

(B) $2\frac{3}{4}$

(C) $2\frac{11}{12}$

(D) $3\frac{5}{6}$

Your Answer _____

_____

Correct Answers

A-70

(A)   First, find the common denominator for the fractions. The common denominator is 12.

$$1\frac{5}{6} \qquad 1\frac{?}{12}$$
$$+ \ \ \frac{3}{4} = + \ \ \frac{?}{12}$$

Now find the numerator that will make $\frac{5}{6}$ equivalent to $\frac{?}{12}$. The new numerator is 10 because $\frac{5}{6}$ is equivalent to $\frac{10}{12}$.

$$1\frac{5}{6} \qquad 1\frac{10}{12}$$
$$+ \ \ \frac{3}{4} = + \ \ \frac{?}{12}$$

Next, find the numerator that will make $\frac{3}{4}$ equivalent to $\frac{?}{12}$. The new numerator is 9 because $\frac{3}{4}$ is equivalent to $\frac{9}{12}$.

$$1\frac{5}{6} \qquad 1\frac{10}{12}$$
$$+ \ \ \frac{3}{4} = + \ \ \frac{9}{12}$$

The next step is to add the fractions.

$$1\frac{10}{12}$$
$$+ \ \ \frac{9}{12}$$
$$\overline{\ 1\frac{19}{12}\ }$$

$\frac{19}{12}$ is an improper fraction. Change it to a mixed number: $1\frac{7}{12}$.

Add the new mixed number to the whole number.

$$1 + 1\frac{7}{12} = 2\frac{7}{12}$$

$2\frac{7}{12}$ cannot be reduced.

Questions

Q–71

Factor the following expression: $x^2 - 10x + 25$.

(A) $(x - 5x)(x - 5)$

(B) $(x - 10)(x + 25)$

(C) $(x - 5)(x - 5)$

(D) $(x + 5)(x + 5)$

Your Answer _____

Q–72

Candace took an exam. There were 75 questions on the exam. If she received an 80%, how many questions did Candace answer correctly?

(A)   60

(B)   64

(C)   66

(D)   68

Your Answer _____

Correct Answers

A–71

(C) The first term in both sets of parentheses must be x in order to have x^2.

$$(x \pm \_)(x \pm \_)$$

The second terms in both sets of parentheses must have a sum of -10 and a product of 25. So the second terms must be -5 and -5.

$$(x - 5)(x - 5)$$

A–72

(A) 0.80 is equivalent to 80%. Multiply the percentage of questions answered correctly (80%) by the total number of questions on the exam (75).

$$0.80 \times 75 = 60$$

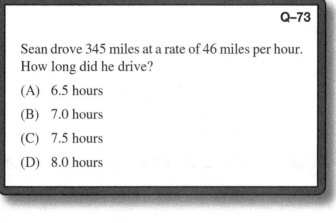

Q-73

Sean drove 345 miles at a rate of 46 miles per hour. How long did he drive?

(A) 6.5 hours

(B) 7.0 hours

(C) 7.5 hours

(D) 8.0 hours

Your Answer _____

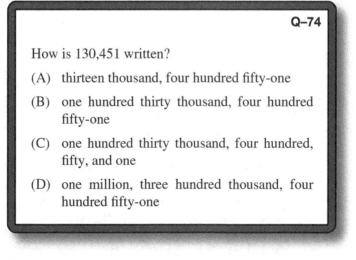

Q-74

How is 130,451 written?

(A) thirteen thousand, four hundred fifty-one

(B) one hundred thirty thousand, four hundred fifty-one

(C) one hundred thirty thousand, four hundred, fifty, and one

(D) one million, three hundred thousand, four hundred fifty-one

Your Answer _____

Correct Answers

A–73

(C) To find the amount of time Sean drove, set up an equation.

$$\text{Distance} = \text{Rate} \times \text{Time}$$
$$345 \text{ miles} = (46 \text{ miles per hour})(x)$$
$$345 = 46x$$
$$7.5 = x$$

A–74

(B) One hundred thirty thousand, four hundred fifty-one is shown as "130,451." Thirteen thousand, four hundred fifty-one is shown as "13,451." One hundred thirty thousand, four hundred, fifty, and one is written incorrectly; there are two unnecessary commas and "and" is used to signify a decimal point. One million, three hundred thousand, four hundred fifty-one is shown as "1,300,451."

Questions

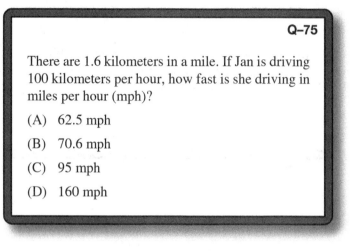

Q-75

There are 1.6 kilometers in a mile. If Jan is driving 100 kilometers per hour, how fast is she driving in miles per hour (mph)?

(A) 62.5 mph

(B) 70.6 mph

(C) 95 mph

(D) 160 mph

Your Answer _____

_____

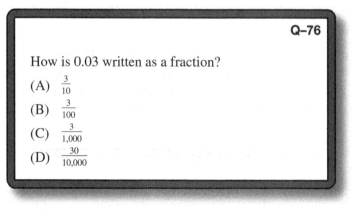

Q-76

How is 0.03 written as a fraction?

(A) $\frac{3}{10}$

(B) $\frac{3}{100}$

(C) $\frac{3}{1,000}$

(D) $\frac{30}{10,000}$

Your Answer _____

_____

Correct Answers

A–75

(A) There are 1.6 kilometers in a mile. 100 kilometers per hour divided by 1.6 kilometers in a mile is 62.5 miles per hour.

A–76

(B) 0.03, or three hundredths, is written as $\frac{3}{100}$. $\frac{3}{10}$, or three tenths, is equivalent to 0.3. $\frac{3}{1,000}$, or three thousandths, is equivalent to 0.003. $\frac{30}{100}$, or thirty hundredths, is equivalent to 0.3.

Questions

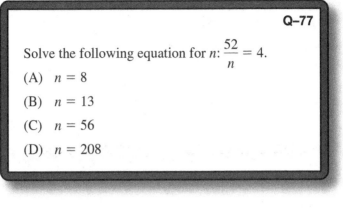

Q–77

Solve the following equation for n: $\dfrac{52}{n} = 4$.

(A) $n = 8$

(B) $n = 13$

(C) $n = 56$

(D) $n = 208$

Your Answer _____

_____

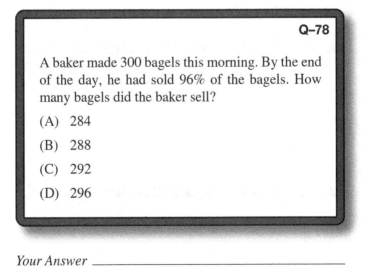

Q–78

A baker made 300 bagels this morning. By the end of the day, he had sold 96% of the bagels. How many bagels did the baker sell?

(A) 284

(B) 288

(C) 292

(D) 296

Your Answer _____

_____

Correct Answers

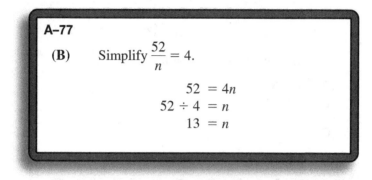

A–77

(B)   Simplify $\dfrac{52}{n} = 4$.

$$52 = 4n$$
$$52 \div 4 = n$$
$$13 = n$$

A–78

(B)   0.96 is the decimal equivalent of 96%. 300 multiplied by 0.96 is 288.

Questions

Q-79

There are 140 students in Professor O'Neil's class. 100 of the students are male and 40 are female. What is the ratio of male students to female students in Professor O'Neil's class?

(A) 2:1

(B) 5:2

(C) 40:140

(D) 140:40

Your Answer ⸺⸺⸺⸺⸺⸺⸺⸺⸺

⸺⸺⸺⸺⸺⸺⸺⸺⸺⸺

Q-80

Solve the following problem: $(-6) + (-7) + (8) + (-3)$.

(A) -8

(B) -2

(C) 2

(D) 8

Your Answer ⸺⸺⸺⸺⸺⸺⸺⸺⸺

⸺⸺⸺⸺⸺⸺⸺⸺⸺⸺

Correct Answers

A–79

(B)   There are 100 male students and 40 female students. 100:40 can be simplified by dividing each side of the ratio by 20, resulting in a ratio of 5:2.

A–80

(A)   First add all of the negative numbers.

$$(-6) + (-7) + (-3) = -16$$

Now add the sum of the negative numbers to the positive number.

$$-16 + 8 = -8$$

Questions

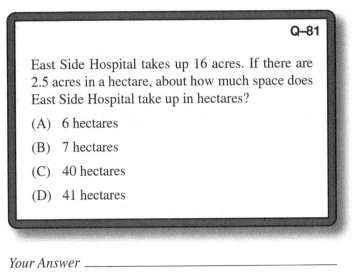

Q–81

East Side Hospital takes up 16 acres. If there are 2.5 acres in a hectare, about how much space does East Side Hospital take up in hectares?

(A) 6 hectares

(B) 7 hectares

(C) 40 hectares

(D) 41 hectares

Your Answer _____

_____

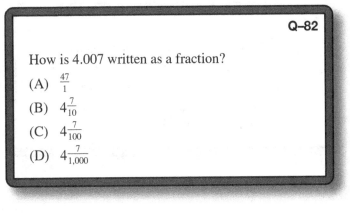

Q–82

How is 4.007 written as a fraction?

(A) $\frac{47}{1}$

(B) $4\frac{7}{10}$

(C) $4\frac{7}{100}$

(D) $4\frac{7}{1,000}$

Your Answer _____

_____

Correct Answers

A–81

(A) There are 2.5 acres in a hectare. 16 acres divided by 2.5 acres in a hectare is 6.4 hectares. 6.4 hectares is rounded to 6 hectares.

A–82

(D) 4.007, or four and seven thousandths, is written as $4\frac{7}{1,000}$. $\frac{47}{1}$, or forty-seven over one, is equivalent to 47. $4\frac{7}{10}$, or four and seven tenths, is equivalent to 4.7. $4\frac{7}{100}$, or four and seven hundredths, is equivalent to 4.07.

Questions

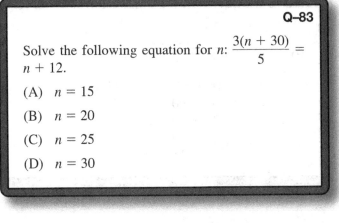

Q–83

Solve the following equation for n: $\dfrac{3(n + 30)}{5} = n + 12$.

(A) $n = 15$

(B) $n = 20$

(C) $n = 25$

(D) $n = 30$

Your Answer _____

_____

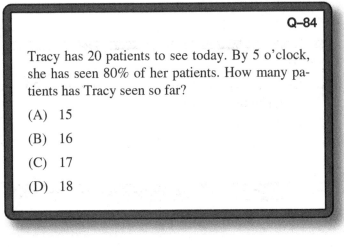

Q–84

Tracy has 20 patients to see today. By 5 o'clock, she has seen 80% of her patients. How many patients has Tracy seen so far?

(A) 15

(B) 16

(C) 17

(D) 18

Your Answer _____

_____

Correct Answers

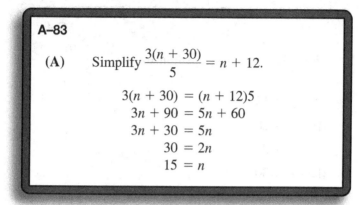

A–83

(A) Simplify $\dfrac{3(n + 30)}{5} = n + 12$.

$$3(n + 30) = (n + 12)5$$
$$3n + 90 = 5n + 60$$
$$3n + 30 = 5n$$
$$30 = 2n$$
$$15 = n$$

A–84

(B) 0.80 is the decimal equivalent of 80%. 20 multiplied by 0.80 is 16.

Q-85

The ratio of students in Professor Kramer's class is 4:3 sophomores to freshmen. If there are 24 sophomores, how many freshmen are in Professor Kramer's class?

(A) 12

(B) 16

(C) 18

(D) 20

Your Answer _____

_____

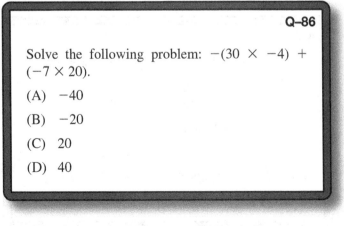

Q-86

Solve the following problem: $-(30 \times -4) + (-7 \times 20)$.

(A) −40

(B) −20

(C) 20

(D) 40

Your Answer _____

_____

Correct Answers

A–85

(C)   Set up a ratio.

$$\frac{4}{3} = \frac{24 \text{ sophomores}}{x \text{ freshmen}}$$

Now cross multiply.

$$(3)(24 \text{ sophomores}) = (4)(x \text{ freshmen})$$
$$72 = 4x$$
$$18 \text{ freshmen} = x$$

A–86

(B)   First, solve the multiplication problems in the parentheses.

$$-(-120) + (-140)$$

Next, $-(-120)$ becomes 120.

$$120 + (-140)$$

$120 + (-140)$ can be rewritten as $120 - 140$.

$$120 - 140 = -20$$

Questions

Q–87

How many liters are there in 350 milliliters?

(A)   0.35 liters

(B)   3.5 liters

(C)   35 liters

(D)   350,000 liters

Your Answer _____

_____

Q–88

Solve the following problem: $\frac{7}{8} - \frac{3}{8}$.

(A) $\frac{1}{4}$

(B) $\frac{1}{2}$

(C) $\frac{3}{4}$

(D)   3

Your Answer _____

_____

Correct Answers

A–87

(A)   There are 1,000 milliliters in a liter. 350 milliliters divided by 1,000 milliliters per liter is 0.35 liters.

A–88

(B)   Because both fractions share a common denominator, simply subtract the numerators. The denominator will stay the same.

$$\frac{7}{8} - \frac{3}{8} = \frac{4}{8}$$

$\frac{4}{8}$ can be reduced to $\frac{1}{2}$.

Q–89

Factor the following expression: $x^2 + 2x - 15$.

(A) $(x + 5)(x - 3)$

(B) $(x + 5x)(x - 3)$

(C) $(x - 5)(x - 3)$

(D) $(x + 2)(x - 15)$

Your Answer _____

Q–90

Matt took an anatomy quiz. He answered 21 out of 24 questions correctly. What percentage of questions did Matt answer correctly?

(A) 85%

(B) 86%

(C) 87.5%

(D) 89.5%

Your Answer _____

Correct Answers

A–89

(A) The first term in both sets of parentheses must be x in order to have x^2.

$$(x \pm \_)(x \pm \_)$$

The second terms in both sets of parentheses must have a sum of 2 and a product of -15. So the second terms must be 5 and -3.

$$(x + 5)(x - 3)$$

A–90

(C) Divide the number of questions answered correctly (21) by the number of questions on the quiz (24).

$$21 \div 24 = 0.875$$

87.5% is equivalent to 0.875.

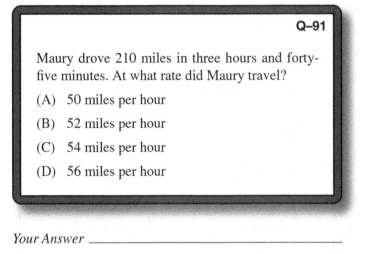

Q–91

Maury drove 210 miles in three hours and forty-five minutes. At what rate did Maury travel?

(A)   50 miles per hour

(B)   52 miles per hour

(C)   54 miles per hour

(D)   56 miles per hour

Your Answer _____

_____

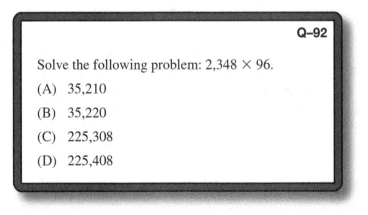

Q–92

Solve the following problem: 2,348 × 96.

(A)   35,210

(B)   35,220

(C)   225,308

(D)   225,408

Your Answer _____

_____

Correct Answers

A-91

(D) First, change three hours and forty-five minutes into minutes.

(3 hours × 60 minutes) + (45 minutes)
$$= 225 \text{ minutes}$$

Then, set up a ratio.

$$\frac{210 \text{ miles}}{225 \text{ minutes}} = \frac{x \text{ miles}}{60 \text{ minutes}}$$

Now, cross multiply.

(225 minutes)(x miles) = (210 miles)(60 minutes)
$$225x = 12{,}600$$
$$x = 56 \text{ miles per hour}$$

A-92

(D) The product of 2,348 and 96 is 225,408. An answer of 35,210 indicates that a 0 placeholder was not used in the ones column and an addition error. An answer of 35,220 indicates that a 0 placeholder was not used in the ones column. An answer of 225,308 neglects to carry the 1 from the tens column.

Questions

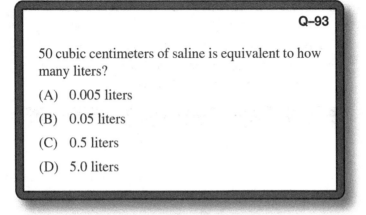

Q-93

50 cubic centimeters of saline is equivalent to how many liters?

(A) 0.005 liters

(B) 0.05 liters

(C) 0.5 liters

(D) 5.0 liters

Your Answer _____

_____

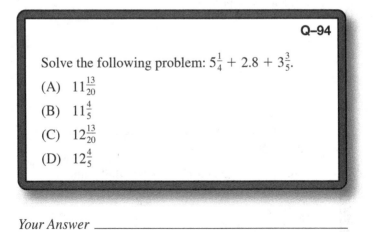

Q-94

Solve the following problem: $5\frac{1}{4} + 2.8 + 3\frac{3}{5}$.

(A) $11\frac{13}{20}$

(B) $11\frac{4}{5}$

(C) $12\frac{13}{20}$

(D) $12\frac{4}{5}$

Your Answer _____

_____

Correct Answers

A–93

(B) There are 1,000 cubic centimeters in a liter. 50 cubic centimeters divided by 1,000 cubic centimeters per liter is 0.05 liters.

A–94

(A) First, change the decimal into a fraction.

$$2.8 = 2\frac{8}{10}$$

Then, reduce the new fraction.

$$2\frac{8}{10} = 2\frac{4}{5}$$

Now find the common denominator for all of the fractions. The common denominator is 20. Then, find the new numerators.

$$
\begin{array}{r}
5\frac{5}{20} \\
2\frac{16}{20} \\
+\ \ 3\frac{12}{20} \\
\hline
10\frac{33}{20}
\end{array}
$$

$\frac{33}{20}$ is an improper fraction. Change it to a mixed number: $1\frac{13}{20}$.

Add the new mixed number to the whole number.

$$10 + 1\frac{13}{20} = 11\frac{13}{20}$$

$11\frac{13}{20}$ cannot be reduced.

Questions

Q–95

Solve the following equation for p: $4(p + 8) = -6(4 + 2p)$.

(A) $p = -3.5$

(B) $p = -2.0$

(C) $p = 2.0$

(D) $p = 3.5$

Your Answer _____

Q–96

Sandra took a final last week. The final had 150 questions. She answered 108 questions correctly. What percentage of questions did Sandra answer correctly?

(A) 72%

(B) 76%

(C) 80%

(D) 83%

Your Answer _____

Correct Answers

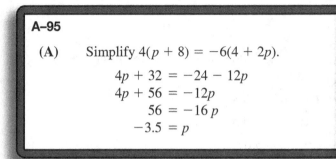

A–95

(A) Simplify $4(p + 8) = -6(4 + 2p)$.

$$4p + 32 = -24 - 12p$$
$$4p + 56 = -12p$$
$$56 = -16\,p$$
$$-3.5 = p$$

A–96

(A) Divide the number of questions answered correctly (108) by the number of questions on the final (150).

$$108 \div 150 = 0.72$$

72% is equivalent to 0.72.

Questions

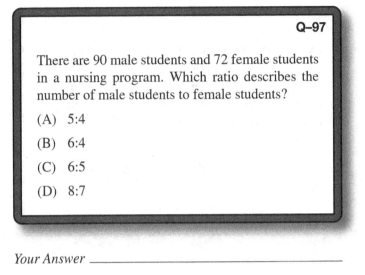

Q–97

There are 90 male students and 72 female students in a nursing program. Which ratio describes the number of male students to female students?

(A) 5:4

(B) 6:4

(C) 6:5

(D) 8:7

Your Answer _____

_____

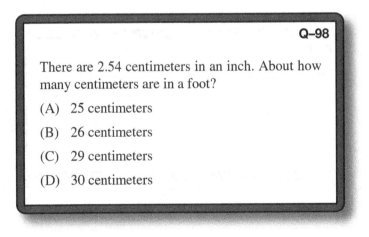

Q–98

There are 2.54 centimeters in an inch. About how many centimeters are in a foot?

(A) 25 centimeters

(B) 26 centimeters

(C) 29 centimeters

(D) 30 centimeters

Your Answer _____

_____

Correct Answers

A–97

(A)   There are 90 male students and 72 female students in the nursing program. This is a ratio of 90:72. Just like fractions, ratios can be simplified. Because both numbers in the ratio are even, you can start simplifying by dividing by 2.

$$90:72 = 45:36$$

Notice that both numbers in the ratio are divisible by 9.

$$45:36 = 5:4$$

A–98

(D)   There are 12 inches in a foot. 12 multiplied by 2.54 is 30.48. 30.48 rounded down to the nearest inch is 30.

Questions

Q–99

Solve the following problem: 97.63 × 2.8.

(A) 97.63

(B) 976.30

(C) 273.364

(D) 273,364.000

Your Answer _____

_____

Q–100

Solve the following equation for x: $5x - 3 = 2(x + 9)$.

(A) $x = 7$

(B) $x = 9$

(C) $x = 11$

(D) $x = 13$

Your Answer _____

_____

Correct Answers

A–99

(C) The product of 97.63 and 2.8 is 273.364. An answer of 97.63 indicates that a "0" placeholder was not used in the ones column. An answer of 976.30 indicates that a "0" placeholder was not used in the ones column and that the decimal was not aligned in the correct place. An answer of 273,364.000 indicates that the decimal was not aligned in the correct place.

A–100

(A) Simplify $5x - 3 = 2(x + 9)$.

$$5x - 3 = 2x + 18$$
$$3x - 3 = 18$$
$$3x = 21$$
$$x = 7$$

Questions

Q-101

Tonya earns $2,850 a month. She spends 34% of her monthly income on tuition. How much does Tonya spend on tuition each month?

(A) $84.00

(B) $750.00

(C) $969.00

(D) $1,010.00

Your Answer _____

_____

Q-102

Felipe drove 270 miles in 6 hours. At what rate did Felipe travel?

(A) 40 miles per hour

(B) 45 miles per hour

(C) 50 miles per hour

(D) 55 miles per hour

Your Answer _____

_____

Correct Answers

A–101

(C)   0.34 is the decimal equivalent of 34%. $2,850 multiplied by 0.34 is $969.00.

A–102

(B)   To find the rate, divide distance by time. The distance driven (270 miles) divided by the time (6 hours) gives a rate of 45 miles per hour.

Questions

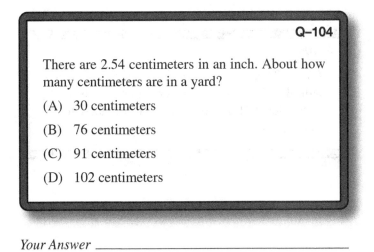

Q–103

Round off 672,458 to the nearest thousand.

(A) 670,000

(B) 672,000

(C) 672,500

(D) 673,000

Your Answer _____

_____

Q–104

There are 2.54 centimeters in an inch. About how many centimeters are in a yard?

(A) 30 centimeters

(B) 76 centimeters

(C) 91 centimeters

(D) 102 centimeters

Your Answer _____

_____

Correct Answers

A–103

(B) The 2 in the thousands place remains a 2 because the digit in the hundreds place is less than 5. The numbers after the thousands place all become zeroes.

A–104

(C) There are 36 inches in a yard. 36 inches multiplied by 2.54 centimeters in an inch is 91.44 centimeters. 91.44 centimeters is rounded to 91 centimeters.

Questions

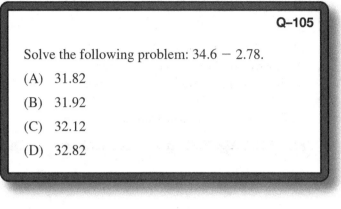

Q–105

Solve the following problem: $34.6 - 2.78$.

(A) 31.82

(B) 31.92

(C) 32.12

(D) 32.82

Your Answer _____

_____

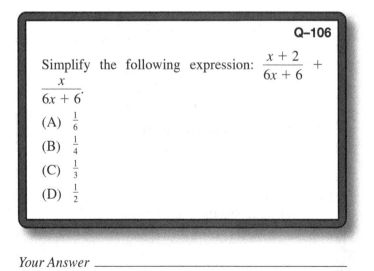

Q–106

Simplify the following expression: $\dfrac{x + 2}{6x + 6} + \dfrac{x}{6x + 6}$.

(A) $\frac{1}{6}$

(B) $\frac{1}{4}$

(C) $\frac{1}{3}$

(D) $\frac{1}{2}$

Your Answer _____

_____

Correct Answers

A–105

(A) The difference of 34.6 minus 2.78 is 31.82. An answer of 31.92 neglects to borrow from the tenths column. An answer of 32.12 indicates a subtraction error in the tenths column. An answer of 32.82 neglects to borrow from the ones column.

A–106

(C) Notice that the denominators in the fractions are the same. Because there is a common denominator, you can add these fractions in the usual way.

$$\frac{x + 2}{6x + 6} + \frac{x}{6x + 6} = \frac{x + 2 + x}{6x + 6}$$

Add the variables in the numerator.

$$\frac{x + 2 + x}{6x + 6} = \frac{2x + 2}{6x + 6}$$

Now factor the expression in the denominator.

$$\frac{2x + 2}{6x + 6} = \frac{2x + 2}{3(2x + 2)}$$

Finally, the expression $2x + 2$ can be divided from the numerator and the denominator.

$$\frac{2x + 2}{3(2x + 2)} = \frac{1}{3}$$

Questions

Q–107

Melissa invested $3,600.00 in an account that paid 12% interest. How much money did she gain in interest?

(A) $380.00

(B) $396.00

(C) $420.00

(D) $432.00

Your Answer _____

Q–108

Lucia drove 264 miles in five and a half hours. At what rate did Lucia travel?

(A) 36 miles per hour

(B) 42 miles per hour

(C) 48 miles per hour

(D) 54 miles per hour

Your Answer _____

Correct Answers

A–107

(D)   0.12 is the decimal equivalent of 12%. $3,600.00 multiplied by 0.12 is $432.00.

A–108

(C)   Set up a ratio.

$$\frac{264 \text{ miles}}{5.5 \text{ hours}} = \frac{x \text{ miles}}{1 \text{ hour}}$$

Now cross multiply.

$$(5.5 \text{ hours})(x \text{ miles}) = (264 \text{ miles})(1 \text{ hour})$$
$$5.5x = 264$$
$$x = 48 \text{ miles per hour}$$

Questions

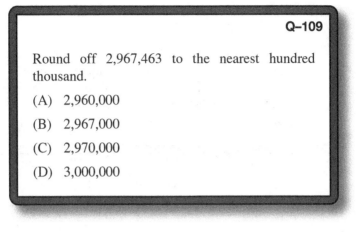

Q-109

Round off 2,967,463 to the nearest hundred thousand.

(A) 2,960,000

(B) 2,967,000

(C) 2,970,000

(D) 3,000,000

Your Answer _____

_____

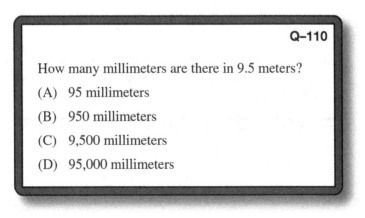

Q-110

How many millimeters are there in 9.5 meters?

(A) 95 millimeters

(B) 950 millimeters

(C) 9,500 millimeters

(D) 95,000 millimeters

Your Answer _____

_____

Correct Answers

A–109

(D) The 6 in the ten thousands place rounds the 9 in the hundred thousands place up to 10. As a result, the 2 in the millions place rounds up to 3. All numbers after the 3 in the millions place become zeroes.

A–110

(C) There are 1,000 millimeters in a meter. 1,000 millimeters per meter times 9.5 meters is 9,500 millimeters.

Questions

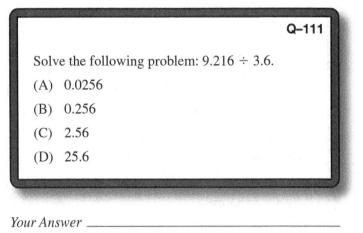

Q–111

Solve the following problem: 9.216 ÷ 3.6.

(A) 0.0256

(B) 0.256

(C) 2.56

(D) 25.6

Your Answer _____

_____

Correct Answers

A–111

(C)   The quotient of 9.216 ÷ 3.6 is 2.56. First, move the decimal point in the divisor one place to the right to make it a whole number.

$$36 \,)\,\overline{9.216}$$

Then, move the decimal point in the dividend the same number of places to the right.

$$36 \,)\,\overline{92.16}$$

Now divide normally.

$$
\begin{array}{r}
2.56 \\
36 \,)\,\overline{92.16} \\
-\underline{72} \\
201 \\
-\underline{180} \\
216 \\
-\underline{216} \\
0
\end{array}
$$

Questions

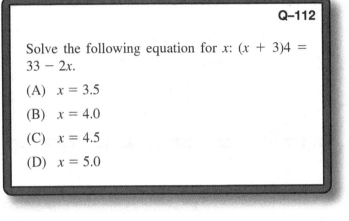

Q–112

Solve the following equation for x: $(x + 3)4 = 33 - 2x$.

(A) $x = 3.5$

(B) $x = 4.0$

(C) $x = 4.5$

(D) $x = 5.0$

Your Answer _____

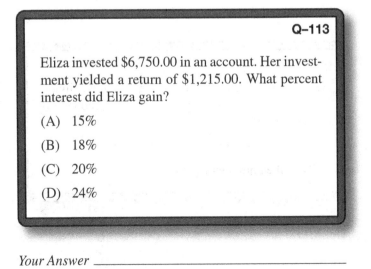

Q–113

Eliza invested $6,750.00 in an account. Her investment yielded a return of $1,215.00. What percent interest did Eliza gain?

(A) 15%

(B) 18%

(C) 20%

(D) 24%

Your Answer _____

Correct Answers

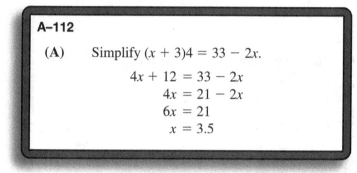

A–112

(A)   Simplify $(x + 3)4 = 33 - 2x$.

$$4x + 12 = 33 - 2x$$
$$4x = 21 - 2x$$
$$6x = 21$$
$$x = 3.5$$

A–113

(B)   To calculate the percent interest, divide the return ($1,215.00) by the amount of money invested ($6,750.00).

$$\$1,215.00 \div \$6,750.00 = 0.18$$

18% is the equivalent of 0.18.

Questions

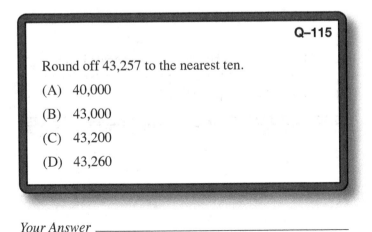

Q-114

The chart below shows the number of sales Cynthia made in six months.

January	February	March	April	May	June
22	18	19	26	17	24

On average, how many sales did Cynthia make per month?

(A)   20 sales per month

(B)   21 sales per month

(C)   22 sales per month

(D)   23 sales per month

Your Answer _____

Q-115

Round off 43,257 to the nearest ten.

(A)   40,000

(B)   43,000

(C)   43,200

(D)   43,260

Your Answer _____

Correct Answers

A-114

(B)   To find the average, calculate the number of sales Cynthia made in six months.

22 sales + 18 sales + 19 sales + 26 sales
                  + 17 sales + 24 sales = 126 sales

Now divide the total number of sales (126) by the number of months.

    126 sales/6 months = 21 sales per month

A-115

(D)   The 5 in the tens place is rounded up to 6 because the 7 in the ones place is greater than 5. The 7 in the ones place then becomes a zero.

Questions

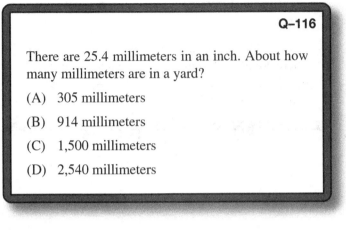

Q-116

There are 25.4 millimeters in an inch. About how many millimeters are in a yard?

(A) 305 millimeters

(B) 914 millimeters

(C) 1,500 millimeters

(D) 2,540 millimeters

Your Answer _____

_____

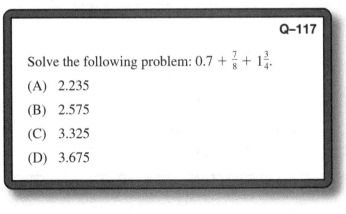

Q-117

Solve the following problem: $0.7 + \frac{7}{8} + 1\frac{3}{4}$.

(A) 2.235

(B) 2.575

(C) 3.325

(D) 3.675

Your Answer _____

_____

Correct Answers

A–116

(B) There are 25.4 millimeters in an inch. There are 36 inches in a yard. 36 inches multiplied by 25.4 millimeters per inch is 914.4 millimeters. 914.4 rounds to 914.

A–117

(C) First, change the fractions into decimals.

$$\frac{7}{8} = 0.875$$

$$1\frac{3}{4} = 1.75$$

Then, add all the decimals.

$$0.7 + 0.875 + 1.75 = 3.325$$

Questions

Q–118

Factor the following expression: $x^2 + 9x + 18$.

(A) $(x + 2x)(x + 9)$

(B) $(x + 9)(x + 18)$

(C) $(x - 3)(x - 6)$

(D) $(x + 3)(x + 6)$

Your Answer _____

_____

Q–119

Cameron invested $8,500.00 in an account. The account lost 15% of its value. How much money is left in Cameron's account?

(A) $1,275.00

(B) $1,950.00

(C) $6,930.00

(D) $7,225.00

Your Answer _____

_____

Correct Answers

A–118

(D) The first term in both sets of parentheses must be x in order to have x^2.

$$(x \pm \_)(x \pm \_)$$

The second terms in both sets of parentheses must have a sum of 9 and a product of 18. So the second terms must be 3 and 6.

$$(x + 3)(x + 6)$$

A–119

(D) First, find how much 15% of $8,500.00 equals. 0.15 is equivalent to 15%.

$$0.15 \times \$8,500.00 = \$1,275.00$$

Subtract the loss in value ($1,275.00) from the total amount invested in the account ($8,500.00).

$$\$8,500.00 - \$1,275.00 = \$7,225.00$$

Questions

Professor Clark's lecture has a mix of sophomores, juniors, and seniors. The ratio of sophomores, juniors, and seniors is 4:7:6. If there are 12 sophomores in the class, how many students are there total in the class?

(A)   39 students

(B)   45 students

(C)   51 students

(D)   64 students

Your Answer _____

_____

Correct Answers

A–120

(C)   Set up a ratio to find the number of juniors in the class.

$$\frac{4}{7} = \frac{12 \text{ sophomores}}{x \text{ juniors}}$$

Now cross multiply.

$$(7)(12 \text{ sophomores}) = (4)(x \text{ juniors})$$
$$84 = 4x$$
$$21 \text{ juniors} = x$$

Now set up a ratio to find the number of seniors in the class.

$$\frac{4}{6} = \frac{12 \text{ sophomores}}{x \text{ seniors}}$$

Now cross multiply.

$$(6)(12 \text{ sophomores}) = (4)(x \text{ seniors})$$
$$72 = 4x$$
$$18 \text{ seniors} = x$$

Now add the number of sophomores (12), juniors (21), and seniors (18).

$$12 + 21 + 18 = 51$$

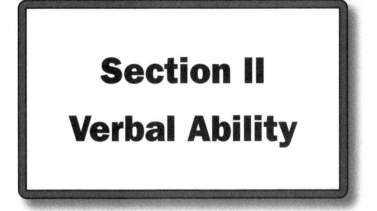

Section II
Verbal Ability

Questions

Q–1

Coalesce most nearly means

(A)   come together

(B)   begin again

(C)   make small

(D)   become thick

Your Answer _____

_____

Q–2

Repudiate most nearly means

(A)   to give up without question

(B)   to scorn as being undesirable

(C)   to reject as having no authority

(D)   to withdraw from consideration

Your Answer _____

_____

Correct Answers

A–1

(A) The word "coalesce" means "to meld" or "to come together," which makes (A) the correct answer. Although the concept of "coalescing" can refer to a process of growth, blending, and changing in shape, which makes (B), (C), and (D) attractive answers, these are incorrect meanings of "coalesce."

A–2

(C) The word "repudiate" means "to reject or dismiss as having no authority," which makes (C) the correct answer. Although the words "rebuke" "renounce," and "retract," to which (A), (B), and (D) correspond, all begin with the same prefix, they do not describe the correct meaning of "repudiate."

Questions

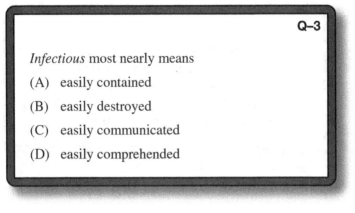

Q–3

Infectious most nearly means

(A)   easily contained

(B)   easily destroyed

(C)   easily communicated

(D)   easily comprehended

Your Answer _____

_____

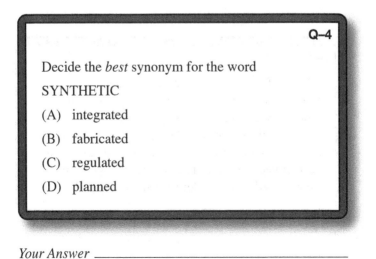

Q–4

Decide the *best* synonym for the word

SYNTHETIC

(A)   integrated

(B)   fabricated

(C)   regulated

(D)   planned

Your Answer _____

_____

Correct Answers

A–3

(C) The word "infectious" means "easily communicated or transmitted." Although some diseases that are infectious may be easy to contain, destroy, or comprehend, options (A), (B), and (D) do not describe correct meanings of "infectious."

A–4

(B) The word "synthetic" means "manufactured," so "fabricated" is a correct synonym. The word "synthesized," which means "integrated" as (A) indicates, resembles "synthetic" but is not a correct synonym. Similarly, (C) and (D) are incorrect because they are respectively synonyms of "syndicated" and "systematized," not "synthetic."

Questions

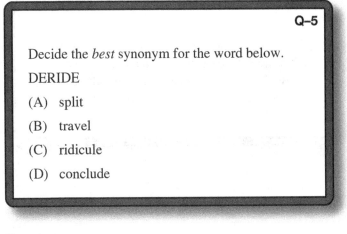

Q–5

Decide the *best* synonym for the word below.

DERIDE

(A)   split

(B)   travel

(C)   ridicule

(D)   conclude

Your Answer _____

_____

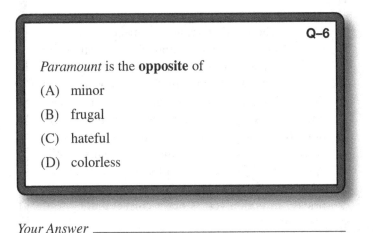

Q–6

Paramount is the **opposite** of

(A)   minor

(B)   frugal

(C)   hateful

(D)   colorless

Your Answer _____

_____

Correct Answers

A–5

(C)   The word "deride" means "to scoff at" or "to mock," so "ridicule" is a correct synonym. Although "deride" resembles "divide," "ride," and "derive," these are not correct synonyms for "deride."

A–6

(A)   The word "paramount" means "supreme" or "pre-eminent," so its opposite is "minor" or "unimportant." Although the word "paramount" contains the word "amount," its opposite is not "frugal," so (B) is incorrect. Similarly, while "paramount" resembles "paramour," which has connotations of love, "hateful" in option (C) is not a correct antonym of "paramount." Finally, while "paramount" is the name of a movie company, which may bring connotations of color film, "colorless" in option (D) is not a correct antonym of "paramount."

Questions

Q–7

Leverage is the **opposite** of

(A) succeed

(B) assist

(C) deter

(D) stay

Your Answer _____

_____

Q–8

Complete the analogy below.

stiffen:relax::

(A) want:desire

(B) study:degree

(C) food:appetite

(D) consider:dismiss

Your Answer _____

_____

Correct Answers

A–7

(C) The word "leverage" means "to build" or "to move forward," so its opposite is "deter." Options (B) and (D) are incorrect because they are both synonyms, rather than antonyms, of "leverage." While the word "leverage" resembles "average," the word "succeed" is not a correct antonym of "leverage."

A–8

(D) "Stiffen" and "relax" are antonyms, so the matching word relationship is "consider:dismiss." In (A), the words are synonyms, which is not the word relationship described in the question. In (B), a degree is something you get after studying, so this is an incorrect word relationship. Similarly, (C) describes an object and the desire for that object, which is an incorrect word relationship.

Questions

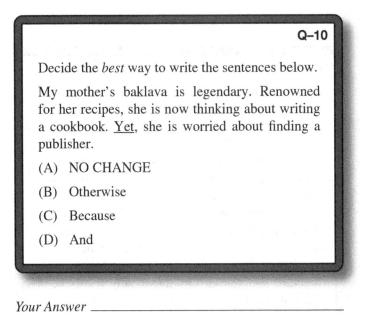

Q-9

Complete the analogy below.

bird:parrot::

(A) mouse:rodent

(B) dog:puppy

(C) cat:catnip

(D) fish:shark

Your Answer _____

_____

Q-10

Decide the *best* way to write the sentences below.

My mother's baklava is legendary. Renowned for her recipes, she is now thinking about writing a cookbook. <u>Yet,</u> she is worried about finding a publisher.

(A) NO CHANGE

(B) Otherwise

(C) Because

(D) And

Your Answer _____

_____

Correct Answers

A–9

(D) A parrot is a type of bird, like a shark is a type of fish. So, (D) is the correct answer. (A), (B), and (C) are incorrect because they do not describe the same word relationship that is in the first half of the analogy.

A–10

(A) This sentence requires a transitional word to show the contrast between the previous sentence and the next idea, which is why "yet" is necessary. (B), (C), and (D) are incorrect because they do not correctly show contrast between the previous thought and the next one. While the word "otherwise" in option B does have a sense of contradiction, it means "on the other hand," which implies the juxtaposition between two opposing ideas that does not occur in these sentences. Similarly, (C) and (D) are conjunctions that connect two thoughts together and also are grammatically incorrect in this context.

Questions

Read the following paragraph.

(1) Last week, I traveled with my friend Taylor to Milwaukee to see our favorite band. (2) However, we were not too sure about the destination. (3) As it turned out, we were completely wrong. (4) The largest city in Wisconsin, Milwaukee is an active place, full of energy and young people. (5) On our first day, we visited the Riverwalk area, which was amazing.

Where is the best place to divide the paragraph above?

(A) NO CHANGE

(B) between sentence 1 and sentence 2

(C) between sentence 3 and sentence 4

(D) between sentence 4 and sentence 5

Your Answer _____

_____

Correct Answers

A-11

(C) Sentence 3 provides a clear end to the first paragraph and a good transition into a new one. Sentence 4 is the beginning of a new idea and requires a paragraph break before it, which makes (C) the correct answer. Options (A), (B), and (D) are incorrect because they do not identify the best place to divide the given paragraph.

Questions

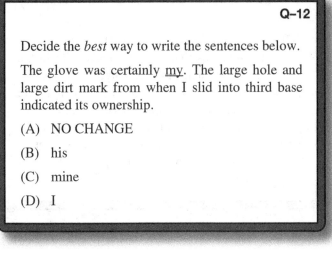

Q–12

Decide the *best* way to write the sentences below.

The glove was certainly <u>my</u>. The large hole and large dirt mark from when I slid into third base indicated its ownership.

(A) NO CHANGE

(B) his

(C) mine

(D) I

Your Answer _____

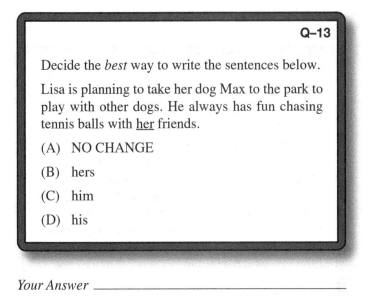

Q–13

Decide the *best* way to write the sentences below.

Lisa is planning to take her dog Max to the park to play with other dogs. He always has fun chasing tennis balls with <u>her</u> friends.

(A) NO CHANGE

(B) hers

(C) him

(D) his

Your Answer _____

Correct Answers

A–12

(C) The use of the pronoun "I" in the second sentence indicates that these sentences are in the first person. As a result, the singular possessive pronoun "mine" is appropriate because it is not modifying anything. Although (B) is grammatically correct, it does not make sense because the passage is in first person. Option (D) is a nominative, singular pronoun that is not possessive, so it is not logical in this context.

A–13

(D) The preceding sentence reveals that this pronoun should be a masculine, singular possessive, which makes (D) the correct answer. If we did not know that Max goes to the park to play with other dogs, then option (A) would be a possible answer. However, this is inappropriate because we have no other information about Lisa's friends. Similarly, (B) is incorrect because it is a feminine, singular possessive. Option (C) is incorrect because it is a masculine, singular, objective pronoun, which does not make sense in the context of this sentence.

Questions

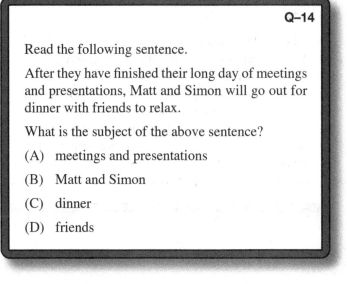

Q-14

Read the following sentence.

After they have finished their long day of meetings and presentations, Matt and Simon will go out for dinner with friends to relax.

What is the subject of the above sentence?

(A) meetings and presentations

(B) Matt and Simon

(C) dinner

(D) friends

Your Answer _____

_____

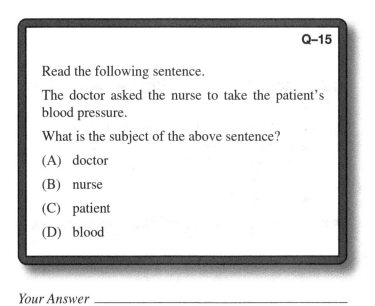

Q-15

Read the following sentence.

The doctor asked the nurse to take the patient's blood pressure.

What is the subject of the above sentence?

(A) doctor

(B) nurse

(C) patient

(D) blood

Your Answer _____

_____

Correct Answers

A–14

(B)   The subject of the sentence is "Matt and Simon" because they are the main source of action in the sentence. While "meetings and presentations" is a noun phrase, option (A) is incorrect because these nouns are not the subject of the sentence. Similarly, while "dinner" and "friends" are both nouns, options (C) and (D) are incorrect because they function to modify the action in the sentence as indirect objects rather than as the subject.

A–15

(A)   The subject of a sentence is the source of action in the sentence, so (A) is the correct answer. Although options (B), (C), and (D) are all nouns, they support the action of the subject of the sentence, which is "doctor."

Questions

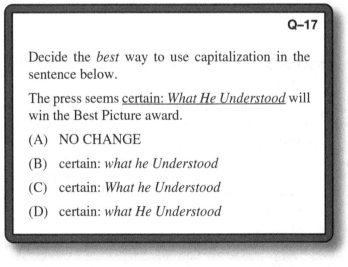

Q–16

Decide the *best* way to use capitalization in the sentences below.

Until I read the article online, I couldn't believe that what <u>Pat told me was true. It was</u> like a crazy dream.

(A) NO CHANGE

(B) Pat told me was true. it was

(C) pat told me was true. It was

(D) pat told me was true. it was

Your Answer _____

Q–17

Decide the *best* way to use capitalization in the sentence below.

The press seems <u>certain: *What He Understood*</u> will win the Best Picture award.

(A) NO CHANGE

(B) certain: *what he Understood*

(C) certain: *What he Understood*

(D) certain: *what He Understood*

Your Answer _____

Correct Answers

A–16

(A) Always capitalize a person's proper name and the first word of a sentence. While option (B) properly capitalizes the name "Pat," it is incorrect because the word "it" is in lowercase at the beginning of the next sentence. On the other hand, while option (C) properly capitalizes the word "It," there is no capitalization of "Pat," so this option is incorrect. Following these options, (D) is incorrect because it does not capitalize either word in the sentence.

A–17

(A) Unless it is done with stylistic intention, the first and last letters of film titles and any other nouns, pronouns, or verbs should be capitalized. In this way, option (B) is incorrect because the first word of the title is not capitalized. Similarly, options (C) and (D) are incorrect because the pronoun "he" and the word "what" are not capitalized, respectively.

Questions

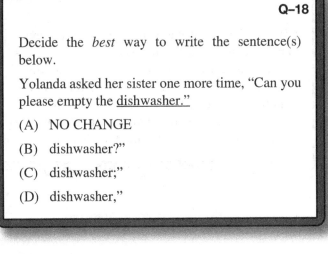

Q–18

Decide the *best* way to write the sentence(s) below.

Yolanda asked her sister one more time, "Can you please empty the <u>dishwasher."</u>

(A) NO CHANGE

(B) dishwasher?"

(C) dishwasher;"

(D) dishwasher,"

Your Answer _____

_____

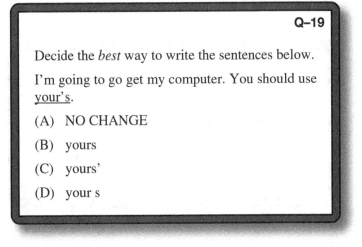

Q–19

Decide the *best* way to write the sentences below.

I'm going to go get my computer. You should use <u>your's</u>.

(A) NO CHANGE

(B) yours

(C) yours'

(D) your s

Your Answer _____

_____

157

Correct Answers

A–18

(B) The use of the word "asked" in the independent clause and the inclusion of the verb before the subject indicates that this is an interrogatory statement or question, so a question mark is required. Options (A), (C), and (D) are incorrect because an interrogatory remark or inquiry necessitates the use of a question mark in this context.

A–19

(B) No apostrophe is necessary in this sentence because this second-person singular possessive pronoun does not require an apostrophe. Indeed, the word "yours" never requires the use of an apostrophe, so options (A), (C), and (D) are incorrect.

Questions

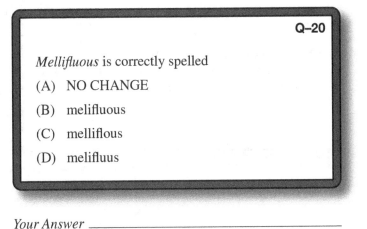

Q–20

Mellifluous is correctly spelled

(A) NO CHANGE

(B) melifluous

(C) melliflous

(D) melifluus

Your Answer _____

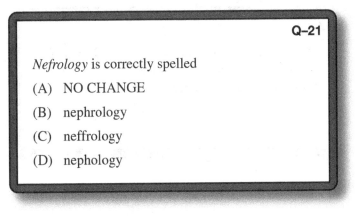

Q–21

Nefrology is correctly spelled

(A) NO CHANGE

(B) nephrology

(C) neffrology

(D) nephology

Your Answer _____

Correct Answers

A–20

(A)   The word is correctly spelled "mellifluous," so (A) is correct. (B), (C), and (D) are misspellings, so they are not correct.

A–21

(B)   The word is correctly spelled "nephrology," so (B) is correct. (C) and (D) are misspellings, so they are not correct.

Questions

Q–22

Incorigibile is correctly spelled

(A) NO CHANGE

(B) incorrigibile

(C) incorrigble

(D) incorrigible

Your Answer _____

Q–23

Jugulur is correctly spelled

(A) NO CHANGE

(B) juggular

(C) jugular

(D) jugalar

Your Answer _____

Correct Answers

A-22

(D) The word is correctly spelled "incorrigible," so (D) is correct. (B) and (C) are misspellings, so they are not correct.

A-23

(C) The word is correctly spelled "jugular," so (C) is correct. (B) and (D) are misspellings, so they are not correct.

Questions

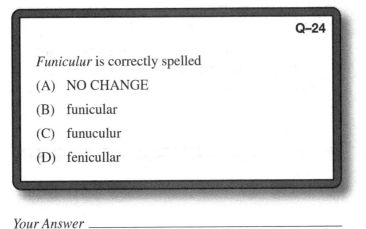

Q–24

Funiculur is correctly spelled

(A) NO CHANGE

(B) funicular

(C) funuculur

(D) fenicullar

Your Answer _____

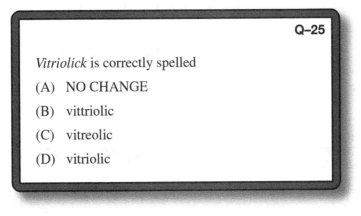

Q–25

Vitriolick is correctly spelled

(A) NO CHANGE

(B) vittriolic

(C) vitreolic

(D) vitriolic

Your Answer _____

163

Correct Answers

A–24

(B) The word is correctly spelled "funicular," so (B) is correct. (C) and (D) are misspellings, so they are not correct.

A–25

(D) The word is correctly spelled "vitriolic," so (D) is correct. (B) and (C) are misspellings, so they are not correct.

Questions

Q–26

Mutable most nearly means

(A) inclined to disaster

(B) capable of change

(C) subject to pressure

(D) related to one another

Your Answer _____

_____

Q–27

Dissolute most nearly means

(A) completely inappropriate

(B) confidently determined

(C) recklessly extravagant

(D) ruthlessly unfair

Your Answer _____

_____

Correct Answers

A–26

(B)   The word "mutable" means "capable of change" or "changeable," so the correct answer is (B). Although the word "mutable" seems like a negative word, which makes (A) and (C) attractive answers, these are incorrect meanings for the given word. Similarly, while the suffix "-able" denotes a relationship between an object or person and an action (i.e., it describes something or someone that is "capable of a certain action"), the word "mutable" does not mean "related to one another." (D)

A–27

(C)   The word "dissolute" means "profligate" or "recklessly extravagant." Although "dissolute" resembles "disappointed" and "resolute," options (A) and (B) respectively do not describe correct meanings of "dissolute." Similarly, while the popular use of "dissolute" in fiction to describe people of ill repute or people who have fallen into disgrace, "ruthlessly unfair" in option D is not a correct meaning of "dissolute."

Questions

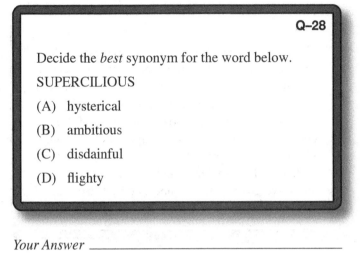

Q–28

Decide the *best* synonym for the word below.

SUPERCILIOUS

(A) hysterical

(B) ambitious

(C) disdainful

(D) flighty

Your Answer _____

_____

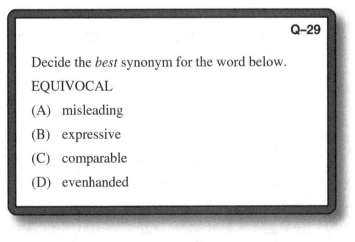

Q–29

Decide the *best* synonym for the word below.

EQUIVOCAL

(A) misleading

(B) expressive

(C) comparable

(D) evenhanded

Your Answer _____

_____

Correct Answers

A-28

(C) The word "supercilious" means "disdainful" or "haughty." While "supercilious" sounds like it might describe a "hysterical" or "flighty" person, which would make (A) and (D) attractive answers, these are not correct meanings of "supercilious." Similarly, while "supercilious" sounds like it might describe the qualities of a superhero or fictional character, which would make (B) an attractive answer, this is not a correct meaning of "supercilious."

A-29

(A) The word "equivocal" means "ambiguous," so "misleading" is a correct synonym. While "equivocal" resembles "vocal," which makes (B) an attractive answer, "expressive" is not a correct synonym for "equivocal." Similarly, while "equivocal" resembles "equivalent" and "equitable," options (C) and (D) are not correct synonyms for "equivocal."

Questions

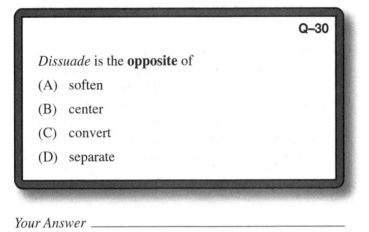

Q–30

Dissuade is the **opposite** of

(A)   soften

(B)   center

(C)   convert

(D)   separate

Your Answer _____

_____

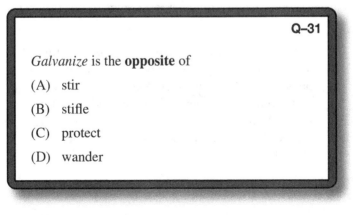

Q–31

Galvanize is the **opposite** of

(A)   stir

(B)   stifle

(C)   protect

(D)   wander

Your Answer _____

_____

Correct Answers

A–30

(C) The word "dissuade" means "to deter," so its antonym, or opposite, is "convert." Although the word "dissuade" sounds like the fabric suede, which makes (A) an attractive answer, this is an incorrect antonym for "dissuade." Similarly, (B) is an antonym of "dissipate," whereas (D) is a synonym for "disperse." So, both options are incorrect.

A–31

(B) The word "galvanize" means "to stimulate," so its antonym, or opposite, is "stifle." Options (A) and (C) are incorrect because they are both synonyms, rather than antonyms, of "galvanize." While "galvanize" resembles "gallivant," the word "wander" in (D) is an incorrect antonym of "galvanize."

Questions

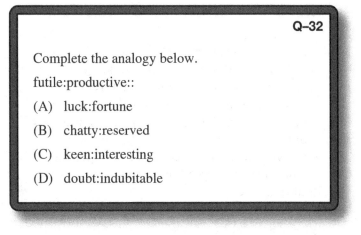

Q–32

Complete the analogy below.

futile:productive::

(A) luck:fortune

(B) chatty:reserved

(C) keen:interesting

(D) doubt:indubitable

Your Answer _____

_____

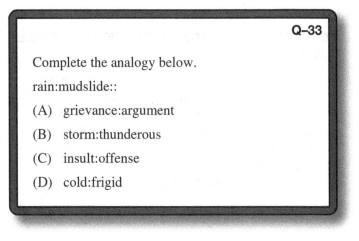

Q–33

Complete the analogy below.

rain:mudslide::

(A) grievance:argument

(B) storm:thunderous

(C) insult:offense

(D) cold:frigid

Your Answer _____

_____

Correct Answers

A–32

(B) The word "futile" means "without purpose" or "unproductive," so "productive" is its antonym, or opposite. As a result, (B) is the correct answer because the words are opposites. In (A), "fortune" is a kind of "luck," which is an incorrect word relationship. Similarly, in (C), the words are synonyms, which is not correct; and in (D), "indubitable" means "beyond or without doubt," which is also incorrect.

A–33

(A) Rain is the cause of mudslides. So, the correct answer is (A) because a grievance is the cause of an argument. Option (B) is incorrect because "thunderous" is a quality of a storm. Similarly, (C) and (D) are incorrect because the word relationships are synonyms of each other rather than having a cause-and-effect relationship.

Questions

Q–34

Decide the *clearest* way to write the sentence below. Note that some parts of the sentence can be removed.

As a young girl, Heather was inspired to be a nurse because she found TV shows about hospitals to be fascinating and interesting.

(A) NO CHANGE

(B) Heather was inspired to be a nurse as a young girl because she found TV shows fascinating and interesting about hospitals.

(C) As a young girl, Heather was inspired to be a nurse because she found TV shows about hospitals fascinating.

(D) Fascinating, Heather was inspired to be a nurse because she found TV shows about hospitals.

Your Answer _____

_____

Correct Answers

(C)   The given sentence, which is included in option (A), is excessively wordy and is not logically ordered. So, option (C) is the correct answer because it is the clearest way in which to reformat the sentence, removing the redundant "interesting." Option (B) is illogically ordered and is also wordy. Similarly, while option (D) removes some of the wordiness, the sentence does not make sense because the elements in the sentence do not occur in a logical order.

Questions

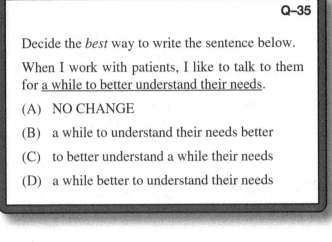

Q–35

Decide the *best* way to write the sentence below.

When I work with patients, I like to talk to them for <u>a while to better understand their needs</u>.

(A) NO CHANGE

(B) a while to understand their needs better

(C) to better understand a while their needs

(D) a while better to understand their needs

Your Answer _____

_____

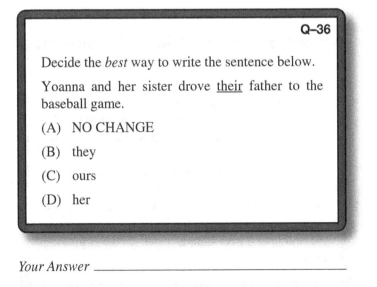

Q–36

Decide the *best* way to write the sentence below.

Yoanna and her sister drove <u>their</u> father to the baseball game.

(A) NO CHANGE

(B) they

(C) ours

(D) her

Your Answer _____

_____

Correct Answers

A–35

(B) Even though some writers utilize split infinitives in casual writing, they are grammatically incorrect. In this way, the correct answer is (B) because the adjective "better" correctly modifies the verb phrase "to understand their needs" in a way that makes sense. (C) and (D) are incorrect because the placement of "better" is illogical in both contexts.

A–36

(A) This sentence requires the use of a nominative, plural possessive pronoun because the sentence begins with "Yoanna and her sister." (B), (C), and (D) are incorrect because they do not indicate the correct pronoun to modify "father." In option (B), the pronoun is nominative but not plural. Similarly, in option (C), the pronoun is a plural possessive but is not nominative; and, in option (D), the singular pronoun is inappropriate given the plural "Yoanna and her sister" in the beginning of the sentence.

Questions

Q–37

Decide the *best* way to write the sentences below.

Sheila asked me to go grab her coat from the coat-rack. When I looked at the collection of coats on the rack, I immediately knew which one was <u>them</u>.

(A) NO CHANGE

(B) her

(C) hers

(D) theirs

Your Answer _____

_____

Q–38

Read the following sentence.

Donna lent Jeff her favorite book for his plane trip to London.

What is the verb in the above sentence?

(A) lent

(B) favorite

(C) book

(D) plane

Your Answer _____

_____

Correct Answers

A–37

(C)   The preceding sentence makes it clear that a singular, possessive pronoun is needed in this context, so (C) is the correct answer. Option (B) is inappropriate because it is an objective pronoun, which does not fit in this context. Option (D) is incorrect because it is a plural pronoun, though the use of the word "theirs" indicates possession.

A–38

(A)   The word "lent" functions to explain the action of the sentence, which is Donna lending her book to Jeff. Option (B) is incorrect because "favorite" is an adjective modifying the word "book." Options (C) and (D) are both incorrect because they are nouns rather than verbs.

Questions

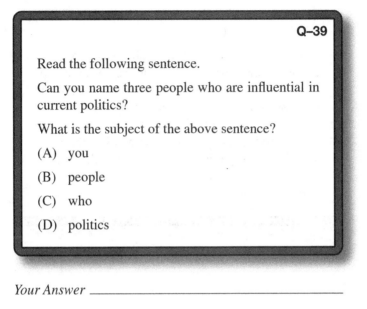

Q–39

Read the following sentence.

Can you name three people who are influential in current politics?

What is the subject of the above sentence?

(A) you

(B) people

(C) who

(D) politics

Your Answer _____

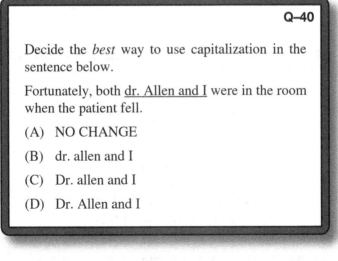

Q–40

Decide the *best* way to use capitalization in the sentence below.

Fortunately, both <u>dr. Allen and I</u> were in the room when the patient fell.

(A) NO CHANGE

(B) dr. allen and I

(C) Dr. allen and I

(D) Dr. Allen and I

Your Answer _____

Correct Answers

A–39

(A)   In this question, the subject is "you" because it is the source of action in the question. Option (B) is incorrect because it functions as the direct object in the sentence. Similarly, option (C) is incorrect because it is a relative pronoun that refers to the word "person." While the word "politics" is a noun, option (D) is incorrect because the word is part of a prepositional phrase rather than the main part of the sentence.

A–40

(D)   Titles like "Dr.," "Mr.," "Mrs.," and "Ms." are always capitalized as a person's formal title. In option (B), while the word "doctor" is not capitalized when it is used to refer generically to the profession, it should be capitalized when it precedes a person's name, as it is a formal title. Similarly, in option (C), a person's name should be capitalized at all times, particularly when it follows a formal title.

Questions

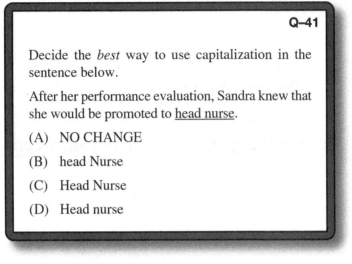

Q–41

Decide the *best* way to use capitalization in the sentence below.

After her performance evaluation, Sandra knew that she would be promoted to <u>head nurse</u>.

(A) NO CHANGE

(B) head Nurse

(C) Head Nurse

(D) Head nurse

Your Answer _____

_____

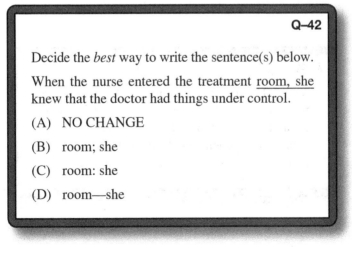

Q–42

Decide the *best* way to write the sentence(s) below.

When the nurse entered the treatment <u>room, she</u> knew that the doctor had things under control.

(A) NO CHANGE

(B) room; she

(C) room: she

(D) room—she

Your Answer _____

_____

Correct Answers

A–41

(C) The context of the sentence indicates that the phrase "Head Nurse" is a formal title, which means that it should be capitalized. Options (B) and (D) are incorrect because they do not correctly capitalize the full phrase.

A–42

(A) The use of the comma in this sentence after the dependent clause is correct. Options (B), (C), and (D) are incorrect because they are not the proper way to connect a dependent clause without an independent verb to the rest of the sentence.

Questions

Q–43

Decide the *best* way to write the sentences below.

Tony likes to chat with his friends on Facebook. But, his girlfriend hates it because she thinks <u>hes</u> addicted.

(A) NO CHANGE

(B) hes'

(C) he's

(D) he s

Your Answer _____

Q–44

Unctous is correctly spelled

(A) NO CHANGE

(B) Unctuous

(C) Untuous

(D) Untous

Your Answer _____

Correct Answers

A–43

(C)   The contraction "he's" requires an apostrophe to correctly indicate that it is a substitute for the phrase "he is." Options (B) and (D) are incorrect because they do not make use of the apostrophe.

A–44

(B)   The word is correctly spelled "unctuous," so (B) is correct. (C) and (D) are misspellings, so they are not correct.

Questions

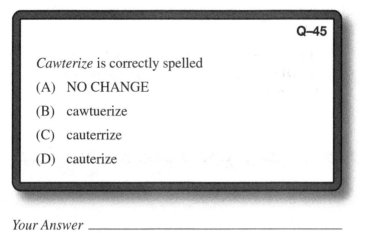

Q–45

Cawterize is correctly spelled

(A) NO CHANGE

(B) cawtuerize

(C) cauterrize

(D) cauterize

Your Answer _____

_____

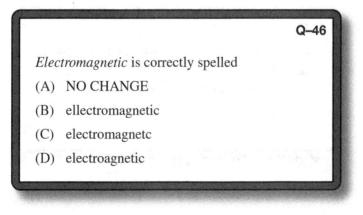

Q–46

Electromagnetic is correctly spelled

(A) NO CHANGE

(B) ellectromagnetic

(C) electromagnetc

(D) electroagnetic

Your Answer _____

_____

Correct Answers

A–45

(D) The word is correctly spelled "cauterize," so (D) is correct. (B) and (C) are misspellings, so they are not correct.

A–46

(A) The word is correctly spelled "electro-magnetic," so (A) is correct. (B), (C), and (D) are misspellings, so they are not correct.

Questions

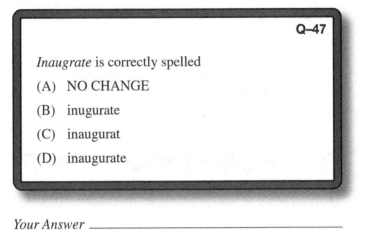

Q-47

Inaugrate is correctly spelled

(A) NO CHANGE

(B) inugurate

(C) inaugurat

(D) inaugurate

Your Answer _____

_____

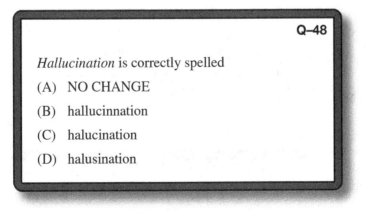

Q-48

Hallucination is correctly spelled

(A) NO CHANGE

(B) hallucinnation

(C) halucination

(D) halusination

Your Answer _____

_____

Correct Answers

A–47

(D) The word is correctly spelled "inaugurate," so (D) is correct. (B) and (C) are misspellings, so they are not correct.

A–48

(A) The word is correctly spelled "hallucination," so (A) is correct. (B), (C), and (D) are misspellings, so they are not correct.

Questions

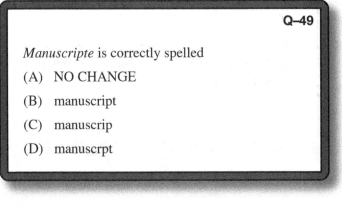

Q–49

Manuscripte is correctly spelled

(A) NO CHANGE

(B) manuscript

(C) manuscrip

(D) manuscrpt

Your Answer _____

_____

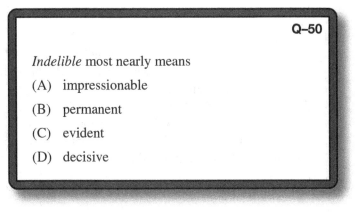

Q–50

Indelible most nearly means

(A) impressionable

(B) permanent

(C) evident

(D) decisive

Your Answer _____

_____

Correct Answers

A–49

(B) The word is correctly spelled "manuscript," so (B) is correct. (C) and (D) are misspellings, so they are not correct.

A–50

(B) "Indelible" means "permanent" or "incapable of being destroyed," which makes (B) the correct answer. Although "indelible" resembles the root of the word "delight," which makes (A) an attractive answer, as well as "decision," which makes (C) and (D) attractive, these are not correct meanings of the word in question.

Questions

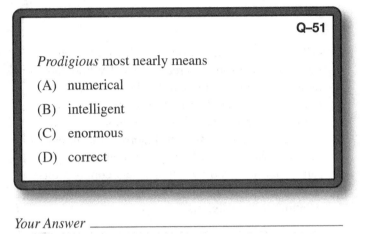

Q–51

Prodigious most nearly means

(A) numerical

(B) intelligent

(C) enormous

(D) correct

Your Answer _____

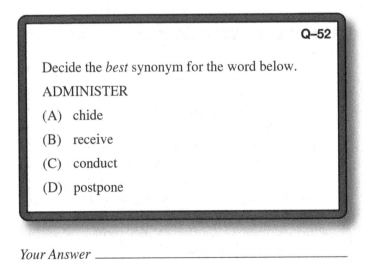

Q–52

Decide the *best* synonym for the word below.

ADMINISTER

(A) chide

(B) receive

(C) conduct

(D) postpone

Your Answer _____

Correct Answers

A–51

(C)   The word "prodigious" means "enormous" or "awesomely great in size." While "prodigious" resembles the word "digit," "numerical" in option (A) is an incorrect meaning of the word. Although "prodigious" is often used as a modifier for "intelligence," (B) is an incorrect meaning of the word. Similarly, while "prodigious" shares the same root as "prodigy," which has connotations of proficiency and exactness, option (D) is not a meaning of "prodigious."

A–52

(C)   The word "administer" means "to conduct" or "to manage," which makes (C) the correct answer. Although "administer" resembles "admonish," which makes (A) an attractive option, this is not the correct meaning. Similarly, while the idea of "administer" as a business concept, such as "administration," may involve oversight of processes like shipping and receiving as well as time management, applications that make (B) and (D) attractive responses, these are not correct meanings of the word "administer."

Questions

Q–53

Decide the *best* synonym for the word below.

CREDIBLE

(A) susceptible

(B) honorable

(C) probable

(D) gullible

Your Answer _____

Q–54

Comprehensible is the **opposite** of

(A) incompetent

(B) admirable

(C) compliant

(D) incoherent

Your Answer _____

Correct Answers

A–53

(C) The word "credible" means "believable," so "probable" is a correct synonym. Although "credible" resembles "creditable" and "credulous," which makes (A), (B), and (D) attractive answers, these are not correct synonyms for "credible."

A–54

(D) The word "comprehensible" means "understandable" or "coherent," so its antonym, or opposite, is (D), "incoherent." Although the word "comprehensible" resembles "competent," which makes (A) and (B) attractive answers, these are not correct antonyms of "comprehensible." Similarly, while the word "compliant" itself resembles "comprehensible," these words are not antonyms. (C)

Questions

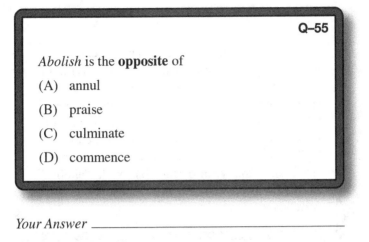

Q–55

Abolish is the **opposite** of

(A) annul

(B) praise

(C) culminate

(D) commence

Your Answer _____

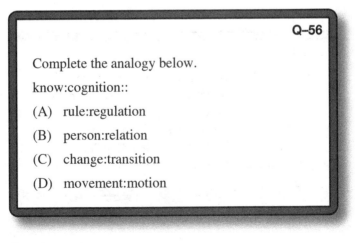

Q–56

Complete the analogy below.

know:cognition::

(A) rule:regulation

(B) person:relation

(C) change:transition

(D) movement:motion

Your Answer _____

Correct Answers

A–55

(D) The word "abolish" means "to eradicate," so its antonym is "commence." Option (A) is incorrect because "annul" is a synonym, rather than an antonym, of "abolish." Similarly, in option (C), while the idea of "abolish" as "getting rid of" something is connected to the act of "culminating" or "ending," this is not a correct antonym for "abolish." Finally, in option (B), while "abolish" can have negative connotations, "praise" is not a correct antonym.

A–56

(C) "Cognition" is the "process of knowing." So (C) is the correct answer because "transition" is the "process of changing." In (A) and (D), the word pairs are synonyms, which is an incorrect word relationship. Similarly, in (B), a "relation" is a type or class of "person," which is not correct.

Questions

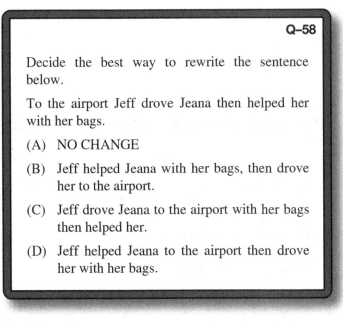

Q-57

Complete the analogy below.

shepherd:callous

(A) nurse:compassionate

(B) farmer:resourceful

(C) bus driver:cautious

(D) police officer:illicit

Your Answer _____

_____

Q-58

Decide the best way to rewrite the sentence below.

To the airport Jeff drove Jeana then helped her with her bags.

(A) NO CHANGE

(B) Jeff helped Jeana with her bags, then drove her to the airport.

(C) Jeff drove Jeana to the airport with her bags then helped her.

(D) Jeff helped Jeana to the airport then drove her with her bags.

Your Answer _____

_____

Correct Answers

A–57

(D) A "shepherd" would rarely be described as "callous" because the term "shepherd" is generally associated with someone who guides people carefully through a certain situation. Similarly, a police officer would not be expected to engage in illicit behavior because it goes against the principles of the job. (A), (B), and (C) are incorrect because they all describe plausible or highly likely adjectives to describe these professions.

A–58

(B) The given sentence does not sequence the ideas in a logical order. Option (B) shows the most likely and logical order in which the events occurred, using transition words like "then" properly. Options (C) and (D) are incorrect because they do not sequence ideas in a logical order, nor do they include the correct transitional word.

Questions

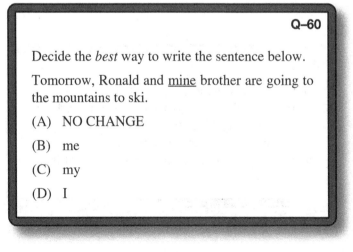

Q-59

Decide the *best* way to write the sentences below.

Kylie is going to nursing school next year. She is looking forward to having a profession <u>which</u> she can directly help people.

(A) NO CHANGE

(B) in

(C) that

(D) in which

Your Answer _____

Q-60

Decide the *best* way to write the sentence below.

Tomorrow, Ronald and <u>mine</u> brother are going to the mountains to ski.

(A) NO CHANGE

(B) me

(C) my

(D) I

Your Answer _____

Correct Answers

A–59

(D) The given sentence, which comprises option (A), is incorrect. In this context, the verb "help" is a phrasal verb, which means it requires the use of "in," and it also requires the use of "which" because a relative pronoun is necessary to complete the dependent clause in which the verb "help" occurs. As a result, the correct answer is (D) because "in which" correctly attaches a preposition to modify "help," which makes the sentence flow logically. (B) and (C) are incorrect because they do not have both elements necessary to make the dependent clause function properly in the sentence.

A–60

(C) This sentence requires the use of a nominative, singular possessive pronoun in order to make sense, so (C) is the correct answer. Option (B) is incorrect because it is an objective pronoun, and option (D) is incorrect because it is not possessive.

Questions

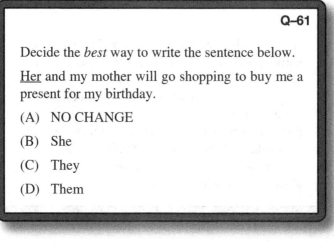

Q–61

Decide the *best* way to write the sentence below.

<u>Her</u> and my mother will go shopping to buy me a present for my birthday.

(A) NO CHANGE

(B) She

(C) They

(D) Them

Your Answer _____

_____

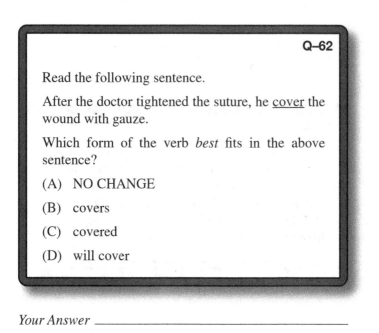

Q–62

Read the following sentence.

After the doctor tightened the suture, he <u>cover</u> the wound with gauze.

Which form of the verb *best* fits in the above sentence?

(A) NO CHANGE

(B) covers

(C) covered

(D) will cover

Your Answer _____

_____

Correct Answers

A-61

(B)   This sentence requires a singular, nominative pronoun to fit the context of the sentence, so (B) is the correct answer. Although option (A) is singular, "her" is an objective pronoun so it is not appropriate. While option (C) is a nominative pronoun, it is plural, which does not make sense in the context of this sentence. Similarly, option (D) is inappropriate because it is a third-person, plural, objective pronoun.

A-62

(C)   The use of "tightened" in the introductory dependent clause indicates that the sentence is in the past tense. So, (C) is the correct answer because "covered" is in the past tense. Options (B) and (D) are incorrect because they are respectively in the present and future tenses.

Questions

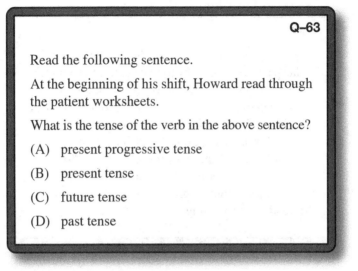

Q–63

Read the following sentence.

At the beginning of his shift, Howard read through the patient worksheets.

What is the tense of the verb in the above sentence?

(A) present progressive tense

(B) present tense

(C) future tense

(D) past tense

Your Answer _____

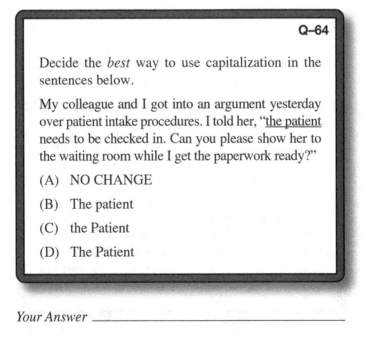

Q–64

Decide the *best* way to use capitalization in the sentences below.

My colleague and I got into an argument yesterday over patient intake procedures. I told her, "the patient needs to be checked in. Can you please show her to the waiting room while I get the paperwork ready?"

(A) NO CHANGE

(B) The patient

(C) the Patient

(D) The Patient

Your Answer _____

Correct Answers

A–63

(D) The word "read" is the third-person singular past tense form of the verb "to read," so (D) is the correct answer. Option (C) is incorrect because the future tense form of "to read" is "will read," which is not the tense of the verb in this sentence. Similarly, option (B) is incorrect because the third-person singular present form of "to read" is "reads," and option (A) is incorrect because the third-person singular present progressive form of "to read" is "is reading."

A–64

(B) The introduction of a quotation with a comma and quote mark means that the first letter of the quotation should be capitalized, as it is an independent thought that is not part of the larger sentence. In this way, option (A) is incorrect because it does not include the correct initial capitalization. Both options (C) and (D) are incorrect because the word "patient" is not a proper noun so does not need to be capitalized in this context.

Questions

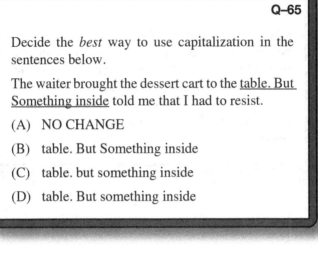

Q-65

Decide the *best* way to use capitalization in the sentences below.

The waiter brought the dessert cart to the <u>table. But Something inside</u> told me that I had to resist.

(A) NO CHANGE

(B) table. But Something inside

(C) table. but something inside

(D) table. But something inside

Your Answer _____

_____

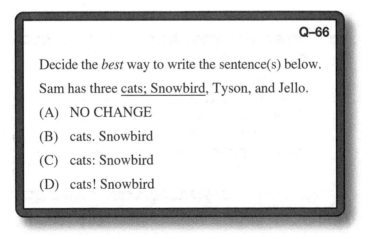

Q-66

Decide the *best* way to write the sentence(s) below.

Sam has three <u>cats; Snowbird</u>, Tyson, and Jello.

(A) NO CHANGE

(B) cats. Snowbird

(C) cats: Snowbird

(D) cats! Snowbird

Your Answer _____

_____

Correct Answers

A–65

(D)   The first word of a sentence should always be capitalized, so (D) is the correct answer. Options (A), (B), and (C) are incorrect because they either do not include a correctly capitalized first word of the sentence or they incorrectly capitalize "something," which is not a proper noun in this sentence.

A–66

(C)   The first part of the sentence introduces a description that is completed by the set in the second half of the sentence. Options (A), (B), and (D) are incorrect because the cats' names do not stand alone as a complete sentence because they are not associated with a verb.

Questions

Q–67

Decide the *best* way to write the sentence(s) below.

The presentation seemed to go on for hours. I am passionate about <u>eighteenth—century</u> history, but her presentation seemed as if it would never end.

(A) NO CHANGE

(B) eighteenth, century

(C) eighteenth-century

(D) eighteenth century

Your Answer _____

Q–68

Cerbral is correctly spelled

(A) NO CHANGE

(B) crebral

(C) cerebral

(D) cerrebral

Your Answer _____

Correct Answers

A–67

(C) Multiple-word modifiers must be hyphenated before a subject in order to be correct. This is particularly true for historical dates and descriptive phrases, such as "twentieth-century technology" or "glass-bottomed boat." In this way, options (B) and (D) are incorrect because they do not correctly set up the multiple-word modifier before the subject of the sentence.

A–68

(C) The word is correctly spelled "cerebral," so (C) is correct. (B) and (D) are misspellings, so they are not correct.

Questions

Q–69

Inclement is correctly spelled

(A) NO CHANGE

(B) incllment

(C) incliment

(D) inclemint

Your Answer _____

Q–70

Plazma is correctly spelled

(A) NO CHANGE

(B) plassma

(C) plasema

(D) plasma

Your Answer _____

Correct Answers

A–69

(A)   The word is correctly spelled "inclement," so (A) is correct. (B), (C) and (D) are misspellings, so they are not correct.

A–70

(D)   The word is correctly spelled "plasma," so (D) is correct. (B) and (C) are misspellings, so they are not correct.

Questions

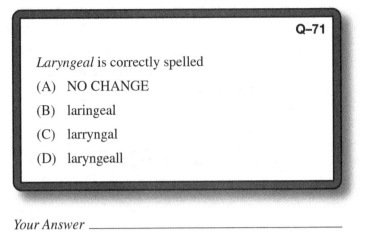

Q-71

Laryngeal is correctly spelled

(A) NO CHANGE

(B) laringeal

(C) larryngal

(D) laryngeall

Your Answer _____

_____

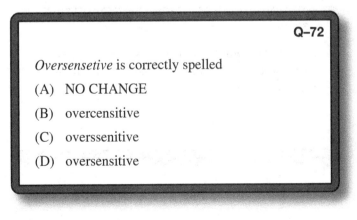

Q-72

Oversensetive is correctly spelled

(A) NO CHANGE

(B) overcensitive

(C) overssenitive

(D) oversensitive

Your Answer _____

_____

Correct Answers

A–71

(A) The word is correctly spelled "laryngeal," so (A) is correct. (B), (C), and (D) are misspellings, so they are not correct.

A–72

(D) The word is correctly spelled "oversensitive," so (D) is correct. (B) and (C) are misspellings, so they are not correct.

Questions

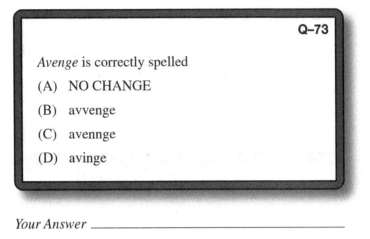

Q–73

Avenge is correctly spelled

(A) NO CHANGE

(B) avvenge

(C) avennge

(D) avinge

Your Answer _____

_____

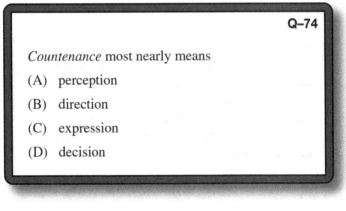

Q–74

Countenance most nearly means

(A) perception

(B) direction

(C) expression

(D) decision

Your Answer _____

_____

Correct Answers

A–73

(A)   The word is correctly spelled "avenge," so (A) is correct. (B), (C), and (D) are misspellings, so they are not correct.

A–74

(C)   The word "countenance" means "look" or "expression," so the correct answer is (C). Although "countenance" seems like it might share a root word with words like "conception," "conduct," and even "condition," which makes (A), (B), and (D) attractive answers, these are not correct meanings for "countenance."

Questions

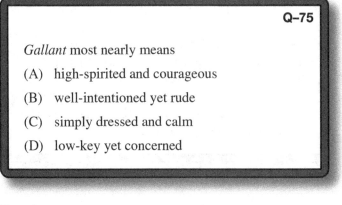

Q–75

Gallant most nearly means

(A) high-spirited and courageous

(B) well-intentioned yet rude

(C) simply dressed and calm

(D) low-key yet concerned

Your Answer _____

_____

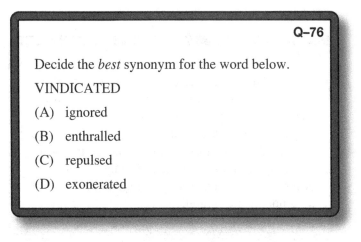

Q–76

Decide the *best* synonym for the word below.

VINDICATED

(A) ignored

(B) enthralled

(C) repulsed

(D) exonerated

Your Answer _____

_____

Correct Answers

A–75

(A) The word "gallant" means "high-spirited and courageous," as in the sentence, "The gallant troops performed bravely in battle." While "gallant" can mean "happy," "well-dressed," or "chivalrous," options (B), (C), and (D) do not describe correct meanings of "gallant."

A–76

(D) The word "vindicated" means "exonerated" or "cleared from accusation of," so (D) is the correct answer. Although "vindicated" seems like a negative word, which makes (A) and (C) attractive answers, these are incorrect meanings of the word. Similarly, while the concept of "vindication" can bring a sense of release or exhilaration, the word does not mean "enthralled." (B)

Questions

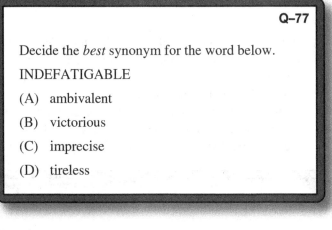

Q–77

Decide the *best* synonym for the word below.

INDEFATIGABLE

(A) ambivalent

(B) victorious

(C) imprecise

(D) tireless

Your Answer _____

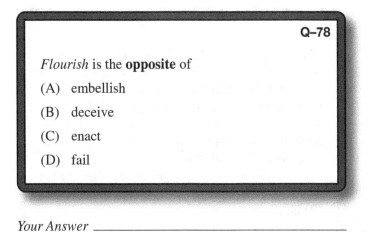

Q–78

Flourish is the **opposite** of

(A) embellish

(B) deceive

(C) enact

(D) fail

Your Answer _____

Correct Answers

A–77

(D) The word "indefatigable," which derives from the same root as the word "fatigued," means "inexhaustible." So, "tireless" is a correct synonym. Although "indefatigable" resembles "indecisive," "undefeated," and "indefinite," which makes (A), (B), and (C) attractive answers, these are not correct synonyms for the given word.

A–78

(D) The word "flourish" means "to prosper," so its antonym, or opposite, is "to fail," which makes (D) the correct answer. (A) and (C) are close in meaning to different connotations of "flourish," so are synonyms, rather than antonyms. Similarly, while the concept of a "flourishing" society might make one think of "corruption" or "deception" as an opposite, this is not a direct corollary to the meaning of "flourish" or its opposite, which makes (B) incorrect.

Questions

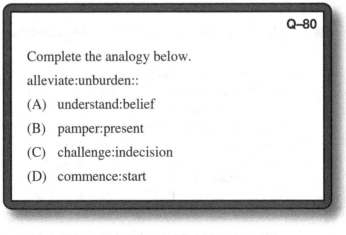

Q–79

Amenable is the **opposite** of

(A) disobedient

(B) responsive

(C) devout

(D) cured

Your Answer _____

Q–80

Complete the analogy below.

alleviate:unburden::

(A) understand:belief

(B) pamper:present

(C) challenge:indecision

(D) commence:start

Your Answer _____

Correct Answers

A–79

(A) The word "amenable" means "accountable" or "manageable." So, its antonym, or opposite, is "disobedient." Although "amenable" resembles "mend" and "amen," options (B), (C), and (D) are not correct antonyms of "amenable."

A–80

(D) "Alleviate" and "unburden" are synonyms, or share the same meaning. As a result, (D) is the correct answer because "commence" and "start" are synonyms. (A), (B), and (C) are incorrect because they do not have the same word relationship as the question. In (A), a "belief" is a concept that one "understands." In (B), a "present" can be the result of "pampering." In (C), the two words are antonyms.

Questions

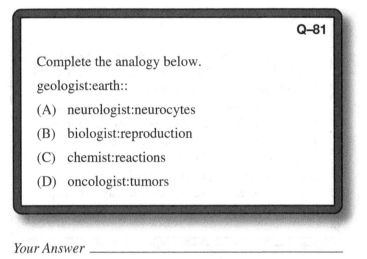

Q-81

Complete the analogy below.

geologist:earth::

(A) neurologist:neurocytes

(B) biologist:reproduction

(C) chemist:reactions

(D) oncologist:tumors

Your Answer _____

_____

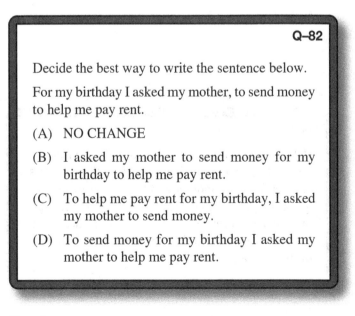

Q-82

Decide the best way to write the sentence below.

For my birthday I asked my mother, to send money to help me pay rent.

(A) NO CHANGE

(B) I asked my mother to send money for my birthday to help me pay rent.

(C) To help me pay rent for my birthday, I asked my mother to send money.

(D) To send money for my birthday I asked my mother to help me pay rent.

Your Answer _____

_____

Correct Answers

A–81

(D) A "geologist" is someone who studies Earth. So, (D) is the correct answer because an "oncologist" is someone who studies tumors. In option (A), while some neurologists may study neurocytes, the general category of "neurologist" describes someone who studies the nervous system. Similarly, in (B) and in (C), while a biologist and a chemist, respectively, study "reproduction" and "reactions," these items form only a small part of their larger study.

A–82

(B) The given sentence needs to be rewritten to have a logical flow of ideas between the subject's request from her mother and the reason for the request, so (B) is the correct answer. (C) and (D) are incorrect because they neither include ideas in a logical sequence nor include correct punctuation of these ideas.

Questions

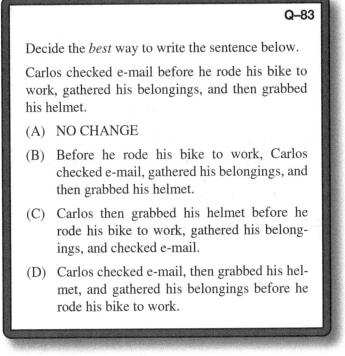

Q-83

Decide the *best* way to write the sentence below.

Carlos checked e-mail before he rode his bike to work, gathered his belongings, and then grabbed his helmet.

(A) NO CHANGE

(B) Before he rode his bike to work, Carlos checked e-mail, gathered his belongings, and then grabbed his helmet.

(C) Carlos then grabbed his helmet before he rode his bike to work, gathered his belongings, and checked e-mail.

(D) Carlos checked e-mail, then grabbed his helmet, and gathered his belongings before he rode his bike to work.

Your Answer _____

_____

Correct Answers

A–83

(B) The prepositional phrase in the given sentence, which comprises option (A), is not in a logical place because it interrupts the flow of ideas. In this way, option (B) is correct because placing the prepositional phrase first is the best way to contextualize the ideas in the sentence without impeding the sequence of ideas in the second half. Options (C) and (D) are incorrect because the prepositional phrase is not placed in the best place and the ideas are not logically sequenced.

Questions

Q–84

Decide the *best* way to write the sentences below.

Ellen received a phone call from a local delivery service.

The delivery man asked, "Hello, may I please speak to Ms. Taylor?"

Ellen replied, "This is <u>her</u>."

(A) NO CHANGE

(B) she

(C) me

(D) my

Your Answer _____

Q–85

Decide the *best* way to write the sentence below.

Before we arrived at the top of the mountain, Jessica accidentally dropped <u>our</u> canteen of water.

(A) NO CHANGE

(B) their

(C) ours

(D) hers

Your Answer _____

Correct Answers

A–84

(B)   This sentence requires a nominative singular pronoun because "is" is a form of the verb "to be," which does not require a preposition. So (B) is the correct answer because "she" is a nominative singular pronoun. (A) and (D) are incorrect because they imply possession. (C) is incorrect because it is an objective singular pronoun, yet no preposition is present.

A–85

(A)   The use of "we" in the first part of the sentence signals that a first-person, plural, nominative pronoun is needed before "canteen" in the second half. Although (B) is a plural, nominative pronoun, it is in the third person so does not fit in this context. Similarly, options (C) and (D) are inappropriate because they are both possessive pronouns.

Questions

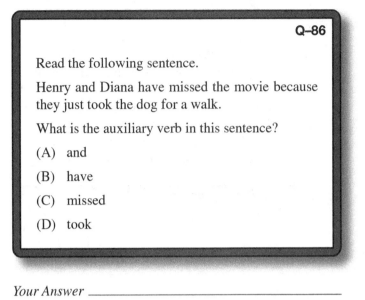

Q–86

Read the following sentence.

Henry and Diana have missed the movie because they just took the dog for a walk.

What is the auxiliary verb in this sentence?

(A) and

(B) have

(C) missed

(D) took

Your Answer _____

_____

Q–87

Read the following sentence.

Luke did not understand how to do his assignment until he received instructions from his teacher.

What is the main verb in the sentence above?

(A) did

(B) understand

(C) do

(D) received

Your Answer _____

_____

Correct Answers

A–86

(B) The verb "have" is used as an auxiliary or helping verb to supplement the main verb, which is "missed." Option (A) is incorrect because "and" is a conjunction, not a verb. Option (C) is incorrect because "missed" is the main verb rather than the auxiliary verb. Similarly, option (D) is incorrect because "took" does not modify another verb.

A–87

(B) The main verb in a sentence refers to the verb that describes the action of the sentence. Since "understand" describes the main action of the given sentence, the correct answer is (B). Option (A) is incorrect because it is an auxiliary or helper verb that modifies "understand." Similarly, options (C) and (D) are incorrect because "do" and "received" modify or support "understand" in the sentence.

Questions

Q–88

Decide the *best* way to use capitalization in the sentences below.

Casey found information for his research paper on climate change at the <u>library of congress in Washington, D.C.</u>

(A) NO CHANGE

(B) Library of congress in Washington, D.C.

(C) Library of Congress in Washington, D.C.

(D) library of Congress in Washington, D.C.

Your Answer _____

_____

Q–89

Decide the *best* way to use capitalization in the sentence below.

Jake prefers to follow current events with online <u>resources; Whereas his friend George</u> prefers to read print newspapers and journals.

(A) NO CHANGE

(B) resources; whereas his friend George

(C) Resources; Whereas his friend George

(D) Resources; whereas his friend George

Your Answer _____

_____

Correct Answers

A-88

(C)   Both "Library of Congress" and "Washington, D.C." are proper nouns and should be capitalized. Although the word "library" is lowercased when referring generally to the concept, both the word "Library" and "Congress" should be capitalized in this context because it is a proper noun as the name of an institution. While the words "library" and "Congress" are frequently capitalized in other contexts, options (B) and (D) are incorrect because both terms need to be capitalized, as they are part of the same proper noun.

A-89

(B)   The use of a semicolon in a sentence necessitates a lowercase letter after the semicolon, unless the word is a proper noun. So, options (A) and (C) are incorrect because they include a capitalized form of "whereas." Similarly, option (D) is incorrect because the word "Resources" is capitalized, which is not a proper noun.

Questions

Q-90

Decide the *best* way to write the sentence(s) below.

It was a quarter to five when Vivien finally made it to the nurse's <u>office, she was</u> worried because she was having trouble hearing after last night's concert.

(A) NO CHANGE

(B) office. She was

(C) office! She was

(D) office: She was

Your Answer _____

Q-91

Decide the *best* way to write the sentence(s) below.

In class, our <u>professor, who</u> is notorious for his asides) spent an hour talking about his new country house instead of teaching us about economics.

(A) NO CHANGE

(B) professor (who

(C) professor: who

(D) professor "who

Your Answer _____

Correct Answers

A–90

(B) A period should be used in this sentence because the sentences represent separate thoughts that are not interconnected. Option (A) is a run-on sentence because each part of the sentence is a separate sentence with its own subject and verb. Option (C) is incorrect because there is no indication of emphasis in the first sentence. Similarly, option (D) is incorrect because these two sentences represent two separate thoughts with a subject and verb each that should be organized into two separate sentences.

A–91

(B) The presence of the closed parentheses after narrative asides means that a single parenthesis must be included before the parenthetical aside. Options (C) and (D) are incorrect because they do not provide the correct beginning punctuation for the parenthetical aside.

Questions

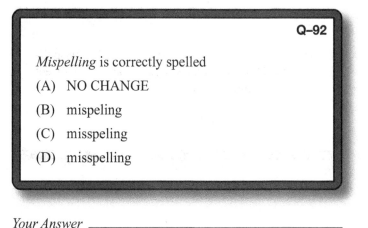

Q–92

Mispelling is correctly spelled

(A) NO CHANGE

(B) mispeling

(C) misspeling

(D) misspelling

Your Answer _____

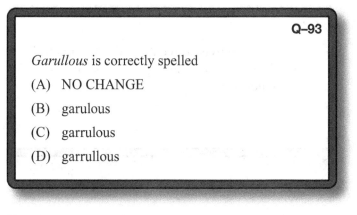

Q–93

Garullous is correctly spelled

(A) NO CHANGE

(B) garulous

(C) garrulous

(D) garrullous

Your Answer _____

Correct Answers

A–92

(D) The word is correctly spelled "misspell-ing," so (D) is correct. (B) and (C) are all incorrect ways of spelling the word.

A–93

(C) The word is correctly spelled "garrulous," so (C) is correct. (B) and (D) are misspellings, so they are not correct.

Questions

Interchangable is correctly spelled

(A) NO CHANGE

(B) interchangible

(C) interchangeable

(D) interchangeabble

Your Answer _____

Stabilise is correctly spelled

(A) NO CHANGE

(B) stabilize

(C) stablize

(D) stabilze

Your Answer _____

Correct Answers

A–94

(C)   The word is correctly spelled "interchangeable," so (C) is correct. (B) and (D) are misspellings, so they are not correct.

A–95

(B)   The word is correctly spelled "stabilize," so (B) is correct. (C) and (D) are misspellings, so they are not correct.

Questions

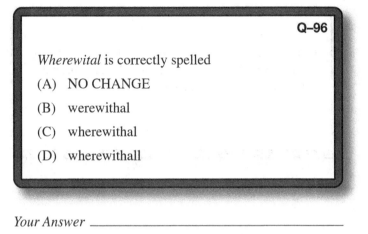

Q–96

Wherewital is correctly spelled

(A) NO CHANGE

(B) werewithal

(C) wherewithal

(D) wherewithall

Your Answer _____

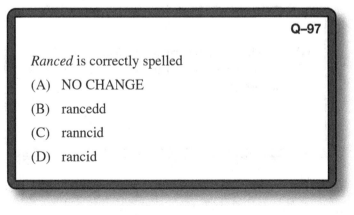

Q–97

Ranced is correctly spelled

(A) NO CHANGE

(B) rancedd

(C) ranncid

(D) rancid

Your Answer _____

Correct Answers

A–96

(C)   The word is correctly spelled "where-withal," so (C) is correct. (B) and (D) are misspellings, so they are not correct.

A–97

(D)   The word is correctly spelled "rancid," so (D) is correct. (B) and (C) are misspellings, so they are not correct.

Questions

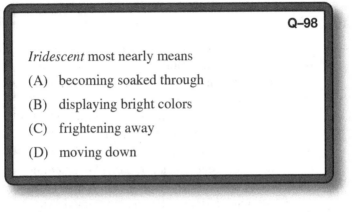

Q–98

Iridescent most nearly means

(A) becoming soaked through

(B) displaying bright colors

(C) frightening away

(D) moving down

Your Answer _____

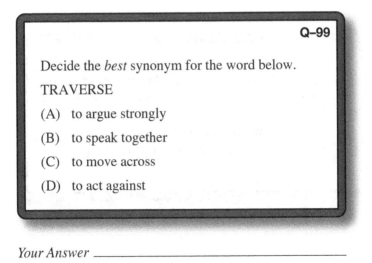

Q–99

Decide the *best* synonym for the word below.

TRAVERSE

(A) to argue strongly

(B) to speak together

(C) to move across

(D) to act against

Your Answer _____

Correct Answers

A–98

(B) The world "iridescent" means "displaying bright colors like the rainbow," so (B) is the correct answer. Although "iridescent" begins with the letters "iri," (A) is incorrect because "iridescent" does not share the same root as "irrigation," which derives from the Latin verb meaning "to water." Similarly, though "iri" sounds like the word "eerie," the word "iridescent" does not mean "frightening away." (C) Also, though "iridescent" contains the word "descent," it does not mean "moving down," as (D) suggests.

A–99

(C) "Traverse" means "to move or travel across," so (C) is the correct answer. Although part of the word "traverse" resembles "converse" and "subvert," which makes (A), (B), and (D) attractive answers, these are not correct meanings of the word.

Questions

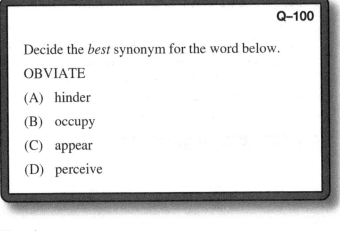

Q–100

Decide the *best* synonym for the word below.

OBVIATE

(A) hinder

(B) occupy

(C) appear

(D) perceive

Your Answer _____

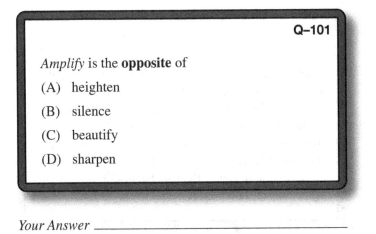

Q–101

Amplify is the **opposite** of

(A) heighten

(B) silence

(C) beautify

(D) sharpen

Your Answer _____

Correct Answers

A–100

(A) The word "obviate" means "to forestall" or "to block," so "hinder" is a correct synonym. (B), (C), and (D) are incorrect because they are synonyms of "obtain," "obvious," and "observe," respectively, rather than "obviate."

A–101

(B) The word "amplify" means "to make louder," so its antonym, or opposite, is "to make quiet" or "to silence," which makes (B) the correct answer. Although the word "amplify" is related to "amplitude," which makes (A) an attractive answer, this is not the correct meaning of the word. Similarly, "amplify" is a concept related to the volume of sound, rather than its beauty or sharpness, so neither (C) nor (D) is correct.

Questions

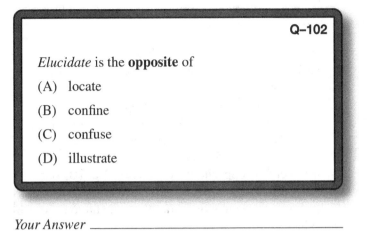

Q–102

Elucidate is the **opposite** of

(A)   locate

(B)   confine

(C)   confuse

(D)   illustrate

Your Answer _____

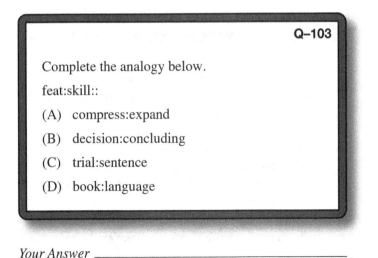

Q–103

Complete the analogy below.

feat:skill::

(A)   compress:expand

(B)   decision:concluding

(C)   trial:sentence

(D)   book:language

Your Answer _____

Correct Answers

A–102

(C) The word "elucidate" means "to explain," so its antonym, or opposite, is "confuse." While "elucidate" resembles "elude," which would suggest an opposite of "locate" in option (A), this is not a correct antonym for "elucidate." Similarly, while "elucidate," which derives from the Latin word *lucidus* for "bright," literally means to "make brighter," its opposite is not "confine," as (B) suggests. Finally, option (D) is incorrect because "illustrate" is a synonym rather than an antonym for "elucidate."

A–103

(B) A "feat" is an "act of skill." As a result, (B) is the correct answer because a "decision" is an "act of concluding." The words in (A) are opposites, which is incorrect. Similarly, (C) is not correct because the two words have a cause-and-effect relationship. In (D), a "book" is composed of "language," which is not the same word relationship as in the question.

Questions

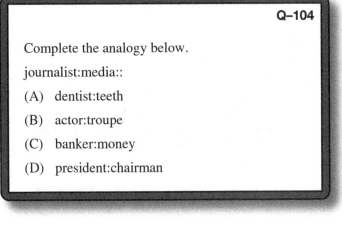

Q-104

Complete the analogy below.

journalist:media::

(A) dentist:teeth

(B) actor:troupe

(C) banker:money

(D) president:chairman

Your Answer _____

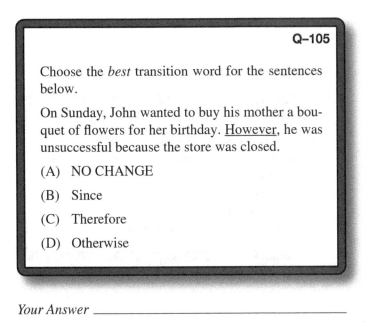

Q-105

Choose the *best* transition word for the sentences below.

On Sunday, John wanted to buy his mother a bouquet of flowers for her birthday. <u>However,</u> he was unsuccessful because the store was closed.

(A) NO CHANGE

(B) Since

(C) Therefore

(D) Otherwise

Your Answer _____

Correct Answers

A–104

(B) A journalist is a member of the media. So, (B) is correct because an actor is a member of a troupe. In options (A) and (C), the dentist and banker both work with teeth and money, respectively, but this is not the same relationship described in the question. Similarly, in (D), a president and chairman both head organizations, yet this is not the correct word relationship.

A–105

(A) The pairing of these two sentences requires an adverb that shows contrast for proper transition between ideas, so (A) is the correct answer. (B), (C), and (D) are incorrect because they imply a causal relationship between two concepts, which is not present in these two sentences.

Questions

Q–106

Decide the *best* way to write the sentences below.

For many years, Detroit has been considered to be the automobile capital of the world. <u>This</u> status is now being threatened as the city faces increased competition from overseas competitors.

(A) NO CHANGE

(B) On the other hand, this

(C) However, this

(D) Also, this

Your Answer _____

_____

Q–107

Decide the *best* way to write the sentence below.

My friends and <u>me</u> went to see a movie last night.

(A) NO CHANGE

(B) my

(C) I

(D) we

Your Answer  _____

_____

Correct Answers

A–106

(**C**)   These sentences require transition to show a contrast between the thoughts of one sentence and the other. So, option (A) is incorrect because transition is necessary. The word "however" is required to connect the thoughts of the first sentence to those of the second sentence while placing an appropriate sense of contrast between them, which makes (C) the best answer. The use of "on the other hand" in (B) implies a sense of corollary or comparison, which is not present in these sentences, so this option is incorrect. Similarly, the use of "also" in option (D) would require the second sentence to be an addition to the first sentence, which is not the case.

A–107

(**C**)   The pairing of the subject "My friends" with "and" requires a nominative singular pronoun. So (C) is the correct answer because "I" is a nominative singular pronoun that fits in the context of the sentence. (A) is incorrect because the word "me" is an objective pronoun. (B) is incorrect because it is a possessive pronoun that does not make sense in the sentence. Finally, while "we" is a nominative pronoun, (D) is nonetheless incorrect because the inclusion of "my" before "friends" indicates that the word that follows "and" must be singular.

Questions

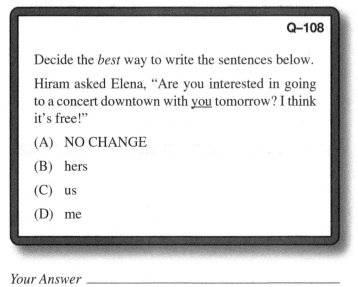

Q–108

Decide the *best* way to write the sentences below.

Hiram asked Elena, "Are you interested in going to a concert downtown with <u>you</u> tomorrow? I think it's free!"

(A) NO CHANGE

(B) hers

(C) us

(D) me

Your Answer _____

_____

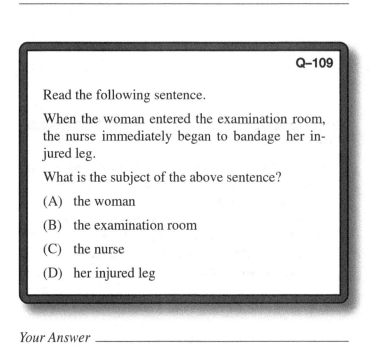

Q–109

Read the following sentence.

When the woman entered the examination room, the nurse immediately began to bandage her injured leg.

What is the subject of the above sentence?

(A) the woman

(B) the examination room

(C) the nurse

(D) her injured leg

Your Answer _____

_____

Correct Answers

A-108

(D) The context of this sentence requires an objective, singular, first-person pronoun, which, in this case, is the word "me." So, (D) is the correct answer. (B) and (C) are incorrect because they are not in the singular first person.

A-109

(C) The noun "nurse" coordinates with the verb "began" to form the basis of the sentence. Options (A) and (B) are incorrect because, while "woman" and "the examination room" are nouns, they are both part of a dependent clause so cannot stand alone. Option (D) is incorrect because it is the direct object of the sentence.

Questions

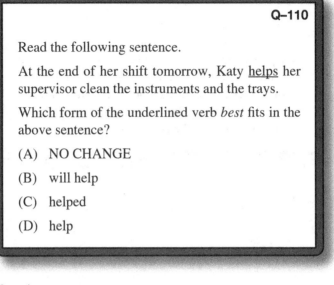

Q–110

Read the following sentence.

At the end of her shift tomorrow, Katy <u>helps</u> her supervisor clean the instruments and the trays.

Which form of the underlined verb *best* fits in the above sentence?

(A) NO CHANGE

(B) will help

(C) helped

(D) help

Your Answer _____

Correct Answers

A–110

(B) The use of the word "tomorrow" in the first part of the sentence indicates that the action is in the future tense, so (B) is the correct answer. Options (A) and (D) are incorrect because they are in the present tense. Similarly, option (C) is incorrect because it is in the past tense.

Questions

Q–111

Decide the *best* way to use capitalization in the sentences below.

Yesterday the book I ordered online arrived in the mail. The book, a mystery story set in <u>the United Kingdom during world war I</u>, is at the top of the bestseller list.

(A) NO CHANGE

(B) The United Kingdom during World War I

(C) the united Kingdom during world war I

(D) the United Kingdom during World War I

Your Answer _____

Q–112

Decide the *best* way to use capitalization in the sentences below.

Joyce's favorite book is *pride and Prejudice*. She admires the confidence of the main character, Elizabeth Bennet.

(A) NO CHANGE

(B) *pride and prejudice*

(C) *Pride and Prejudice*

(D) *Pride And Prejudice*

Your Answer _____

Correct Answers

A-111

(D)   Proper nouns, including the names of countries and major events, are always capitalized. So (D) is the correct answer because it includes capitalization of both "United Kingdom" and "World War I." (A) and (C) are incorrect because they do not include correct capitalizations of both parts of the phrase. Similarly, (B) is incorrect because, though organizations sometimes include a capitalized "The" in front of their corporate names, this does not apply to the capitalization of country names.

A-112

(C)   In a book title, the first and last words should always be capitalized, but conjunctions like "and" should not. Option (A) is incorrect because it incorrectly lowercases the first word of the title. Similarly, option (B) is incorrect because all of the words are in lowercase; and option (D) capitalizes the word "and," which is not correct.

Questions

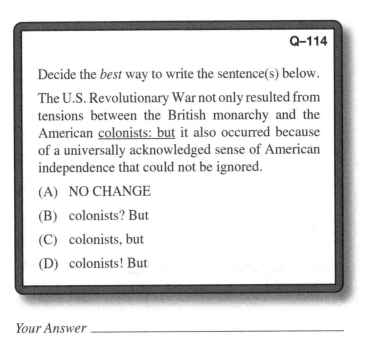

Q–113

Decide the *best* way to write the sentence(s) below.

Long before he became president, George Washington trained <u>as a surveyor and he also was</u> a famous soldier in the Revolutionary War.

(A) NO CHANGE

(B) as a surveyor, and he also was

(C) as a surveyor. He also was

(D) as a surveyor: he also was

Your Answer _____

Q–114

Decide the *best* way to write the sentence(s) below.

The U.S. Revolutionary War not only resulted from tensions between the British monarchy and the American <u>colonists: but</u> it also occurred because of a universally acknowledged sense of American independence that could not be ignored.

(A) NO CHANGE

(B) colonists? But

(C) colonists, but

(D) colonists! But

Your Answer _____

255

Correct Answers

A–113

(C)   This sentence needs to be corrected in order to break the run-on sentence into two separate sentences complete with punctuation and capitalization. So, (C) is the correct answer. Sentences with two separate ideas generally should be split into two separate sentences, rather than being joined by "and" as in (A), a comma as in (B), or a colon as in (D).

A–114

(C)   These two sentences are independent but interrelated with the use of "not only ... but also," so a comma is the correct punctuation in this instance. Options (A), (B), and (D) are incorrect because they do not logically connect these two sentences.

Questions

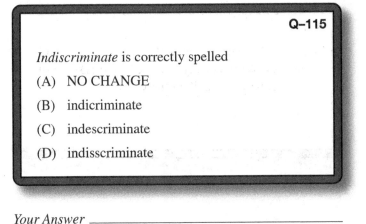

Q–115

Indiscriminate is correctly spelled

(A) NO CHANGE

(B) indicriminate

(C) indescriminate

(D) indisscriminate

Your Answer _____

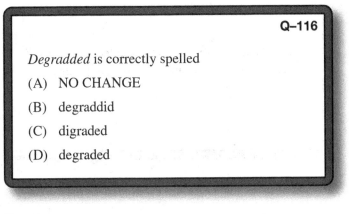

Q–116

Degradded is correctly spelled

(A) NO CHANGE

(B) degraddid

(C) digraded

(D) degraded

Your Answer _____

Correct Answers

A–115

(A) The word is correctly spelled "indiscriminate," so (A) is correct. (B), (C), and (D) are all incorrect ways of spelling the word.

A–116

(D) The word is correctly spelled "degraded," so (D) is correct. (B) and (C) are misspellings, so they are not correct.

Questions

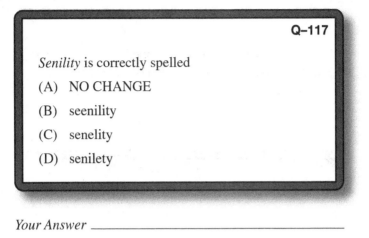

Q-117

Senility is correctly spelled

(A) NO CHANGE

(B) seenility

(C) senelity

(D) senilety

Your Answer _____

_____

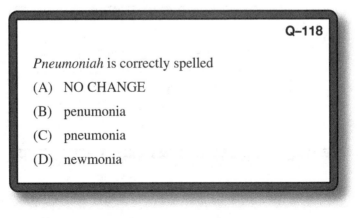

Q-118

Pneumoniah is correctly spelled

(A) NO CHANGE

(B) penumonia

(C) pneumonia

(D) newmonia

Your Answer _____

_____

Correct Answers

A–117

(A) The word is correctly spelled "senility," so (A) is correct. (B), (C), and (D) are misspellings, so they are not correct.

A–118

(C) The word is correctly spelled "pneumonia," so (C) is correct. (B) and (D) are misspellings, so they are not correct.

Questions

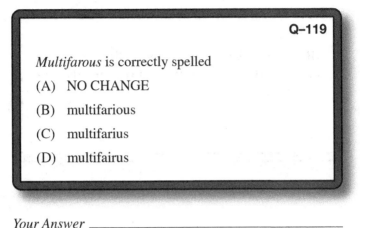

Q-119

Multifarous is correctly spelled

(A) NO CHANGE

(B) multifarious

(C) multifarius

(D) multifairus

Your Answer _____

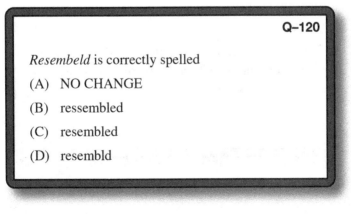

Q-120

Resembeld is correctly spelled

(A) NO CHANGE

(B) ressembled

(C) resembled

(D) resembld

Your Answer _____

Correct Answers

A–119

(B)   The word is correctly spelled "multifarious," so (B) is correct. (C) and (D) are misspellings, so they are not correct.

A–120

(C)   The word is correctly spelled "resembled," so (C) is correct. (B) and (D) are misspellings, so they are not correct.

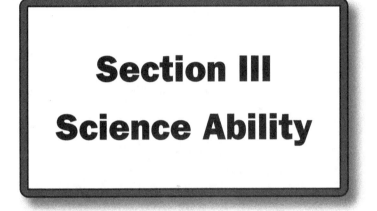

Section III
Science Ability

Questions

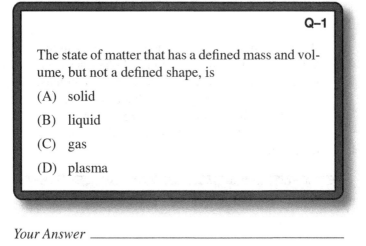

Q–1

The state of matter that has a defined mass and volume, but not a defined shape, is

(A) solid

(B) liquid

(C) gas

(D) plasma

Your Answer _____

_____

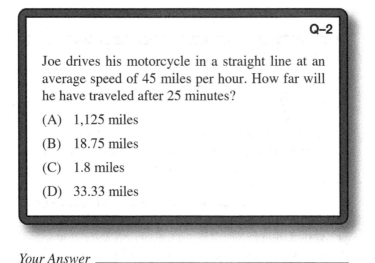

Q–2

Joe drives his motorcycle in a straight line at an average speed of 45 miles per hour. How far will he have traveled after 25 minutes?

(A) 1,125 miles

(B) 18.75 miles

(C) 1.8 miles

(D) 33.33 miles

Your Answer _____

_____

Correct Answers

A–1

(B) A liquid has a defined mass and volume, but not a defined shape. Blood and other body fluids are examples of liquids. A solid has a defined mass, volume, and shape. A gas has a defined mass, but not a defined volume or shape. A plasma is a highly ionized, hot gas that is found in stars and fusion reactors.

A–2

(B) The distance traveled is calculated by multiplying the velocity by the time taken. Because the velocity is in miles per hour and the time taken is in minutes, the time taken must first be converted from minutes into hours, by dividing by 60. Thus, 25 minutes is equivalent to 25/60 hours. If this conversion is not done, (45 miles/hour) × (25 minutes) would give you answer choice (A), 1,125 miles, which is incorrect. By using the converted time taken, (45 miles/hour) × (25/60 hours) you would get the correct answer of 18.75 miles.

Questions

Q–3

Molality is one way of expressing concentration. What is the equation for calculating molality?

(A) moles of solute/kilograms of solute

(B) kilograms of solvent/moles of solute

(C) moles of solute/moles of solvent

(D) moles of solute/kilograms of solvent

Your Answer _____

_____

Q–4

In humans, attached earlobes (E) are dominant to unattached earlobes (e). What is the chance that a heterozygous male and an unattached earlobe female will produce a child with attached earlobes?

(A) 100%

(B) 50%

(C) 25%

(D) 0%

Your Answer _____

_____

Correct Answers

A-3

(D) The equation for calculating molality is moles of solute/kilograms of solvent. None of the other choices reflect the correct equation. Molality is sometimes confused with molarity. While molarity is defined as moles of solute that are in a liter of solution, molality is moles of solution per kilogram of solvent.

A-4

(B) Recall that each parent contributes half of each genetic trait to the offspring, or one allele. Set up a Punnett square with the parental genotypes heterozygous male (Ee) and recessive female (ee). Solving this Punnett square will yield the following possibilities for offspring: 50% Ee and 50% ee. Since only the Ee genotype represents the dominant attached earlobe trait, the correct answer is 50%.

Questions

Q–5

In photosynthesis, light strikes which molecule and releases high-energy electrons and protons, leading to the process of chemiosmotic phosphorylation?

(A)   water

(B)   glucose

(C)   carbon dioxide

(D)   oxygen

Your Answer _____

_____

Q–6

If helium gas at 100 mmHg in a 1-liter flask is forced into a 1-liter flask containing hydrogen at 200 mmHg, what is the pressure of the new mixture?

(A)   50 mmHg

(B)   100 mmHg

(C)   200 mmHg

(D)   300 mmHg

Your Answer _____

_____

Correct Answers

A–5

(A) Water is the correct answer. Light strikes water during the light reactions of photosynthesis, producing high-energy electrons and protons and the waste product of oxygen. The other answers are incorrect.

A–6

(D) If 1 liter of helium gas at 100 mmHg is forced into a 1-liter flask of hydrogen gas at 200 mmHg, the pressure of the new mixture will be 300 mmHg. This follows Dalton's law of partial pressures, which states that the sum of the partial pressures of all the different gases in a mixture is equal to the total pressure of the mixture. 50 mmHg, 100 mmHg, and 200 mmHg are all below the sum of the pressures of the two gases in this mixture.

Questions

Q–7

A firefighter with a mass of 85 kg slides down a vertical pole, accelerating at 3 m/s². The force of friction that acts on the firefighter is

(A)   28.3 N

(B)   255.0 N

(C)   578.9 N

(D)   833.9 N

Your Answer _____

_____

Q–8

The microscopic structures of the kidney responsible for filtering the blood are called

(A)   renal pyramids

(B)   nephrons

(C)   flame cells

(D)   ureters

Your Answer _____

_____

Correct Answers

A–7

(C) Free-fall acceleration due to gravity is 9.81 m/s². Since the firefighter's acceleration is only 3 m/s², the force of friction on the pole slows the firefighter by 6.81 m/s². Force is defined as mass multiplied by acceleration.

$$F = ma$$
$$F = (85 \text{ kg})(6.81 \text{ m/s}^2)$$
$$F = 578.9 \text{ N}$$

A–8

(B) Nephrons is the correct answer. Nephrons are the most basic structure of the kidney and are responsible for filtering blood and removing waste products. (A) Each kidney contains several cone-shaped sections called renal pyramids. (C) Flame cells are the most basic excretory system structure and are found in flatworms. (D) The ureter is a tube that transports urine from the kidney to the bladder.

Questions

Q-9

If you know the pressure of a gas, which three other variables are needed to approximate the moles of gas present?

(A)   volume and temperature

(B)   volume and chemical formula

(C)   temperature and density

(D)   temperature and chemical formula

Your Answer _____

_____

Correct Answers

A–9

(A) Volume and temperature are the variables needed to approximate the moles of gas present if you already know the pressure of a gas. The ideal gas law can be defined by the equation $PV = nRT$, where P is pressure, V is volume, n is the number of moles, R is the gas constant, and T is temperature. R is the only factor that is not a variable; it is always held steady at 8.314 joules/kelvin.

Questions

Q–10

A volleyball, which weighs 2,200 grams, is raised 180 centimeters above the ground. What is the gravitational potential energy of the volleyball?

(A)   3,884,760 J

(B)   38,847.60 J

(C)   3,884.76 J

(D)   38.85 J

Your Answer _____

_____

Correct Answers

A–10

(D)   Potential energy is stored energy, or in other words, the amount of energy that an object could have should it move from one place to another. Gravitational potential energy is the amount of stored energy that an object has due to the position relative to a gravitational source. Gravitational potential energy is defined as:

$$PE_g = mgh$$

Gravitational Potential Energy = Mass × Free-fall Acceleration × Height

In this case, the gravitational pull is coming from Earth, which has a free-fall acceleration of 9.81 m/s². The standard unit of measure for potential energy is the joule, which has units of kg · m²/s². Because of this standard unit, before any calculations can be done, the mass of the object, 2,200 grams, needs to be converted to 2.2 kilograms. Likewise, the 180 centimeters needs to be converted to 1.8 meters. The gravitational potential energy can then be calculated:

$$PE_g = (2.2 \text{ kg})(9.81 \text{ m/s}^2)(1.8 \text{ m})$$
$$PE_g = 38.85 \text{ J}$$

Questions

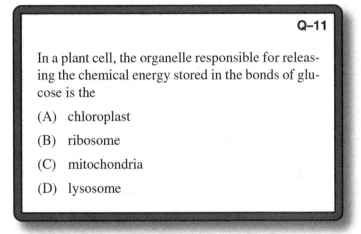

Q–11

In a plant cell, the organelle responsible for releasing the chemical energy stored in the bonds of glucose is the

(A) chloroplast

(B) ribosome

(C) mitochondria

(D) lysosome

Your Answer _____

_____

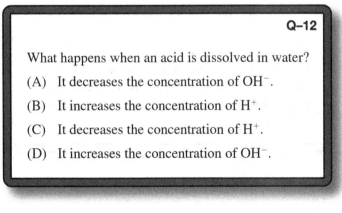

Q–12

What happens when an acid is dissolved in water?

(A) It decreases the concentration of OH^-.

(B) It increases the concentration of H^+.

(C) It decreases the concentration of H^+.

(D) It increases the concentration of OH^-.

Your Answer _____

_____

Correct Answers

A-11

(C) Whether in a plant or animal cell, the mitochondria are responsible for releasing the chemical energy of glucose through the process of cellular respiration. Chloroplasts capture the sun's energy and store it in the chemical bonds of glucose. Ribosomes are responsible for the translation of mRNA into protein. Lysosomes are sac-like vesicles full of digestive enzymes responsible for breaking up food substances in cells and apoptosis.

A-12

(B) An acid is a substance that, when dissolved in water, increases the concentration of H^+. A base dissolved in water increases the concentration of OH^-. Decreasing H^+ or OH^- does not define an acid or a base.

Questions

Q–13

A convex spherical mirror will make an image appear

(A) upright and smaller

(B) upright and larger

(C) upside down and smaller

(D) upside down and larger

Your Answer _____

Q–14

Which of the following organic molecules represent a reactant for cellular respiration?

(A) carbohydrates

(B) nucleic acids

(C) phospholipids

(D) amino acids

Your Answer _____

Correct Answers

A–13

(A)   Unlike the flat mirror on the driver's side of a car, which produces unmagnified images, the passenger side mirror of most recent-model cars has a convex spherical mirror. This means that the mirror bulges slightly outward at the center. This type of mirror is also called a diverging mirror because the incoming rays diverge after reflection as though they were coming from some point behind the mirror. For this reason the reflected image always appears upright and smaller than the actual object. This is the reason that most passenger side mirrors carry the warning, "objects are closer than they appear."

A–14

(A)   Carbohydrates is the correct answer. The reactants for cellular respiration are glucose, a carbohydrate, and oxygen. None of the other choices are part of the cellular respiration equation. (B) Nucleic acids are the informational storage component of DNA. (C) Phospholipids are part of the sugar phosphate backbone of the DNA molecule. (D) Amino acids are the building blocks of proteins.

Questions

Q–15

The strengths of acids and bases are ranked according to their pH, which is the concentration of the hydrogen ion (H^4). What substance has a neutral pH of 7.0?

(A) lemon juice

(B) urine

(C) water

(D) baking soda

Your Answer _____

_____

Q–16

A 1,620 kg car has a forward applied force of 4,250 N. The car is experiencing an air resistance force of 1,160 N. What is the car's acceleration?

(A) 0.5 m/s²

(B) 1.9 m/s²

(C) 2.6 m/s²

(D) 3.3 m/s²

Your Answer _____

_____

Correct Answers

A-15

(C) Water is well known for having a neutral pH of 7.0. Lemon juice is acidic, with a pH of about 2. Urine is also acidic, with a pH of about 5. Bleach is basic, with a pH of about 12.

A-16

(B) Newton's second law states that the acceleration of an object is directly proportional to the new external force acting on the object and inversely proportional to the object's mass.

$$\Sigma F = ma$$
Net External Force = Mass × Acceleration

Rearranging this equation to solve for acceleration:

$$a = \Sigma F / m$$

The net external force of the car is the forward applied force minus the air resistance that is pushing against the car in the opposite direction:

$$\Sigma F = 4{,}250 \text{ N} - 1{,}160 \text{ N} = 3{,}090 \text{ N}$$
$$a = 3{,}090 \text{ N} / 1{,}620 \text{ kg} = 1.9 \text{ m/s}^2$$

Questions

Q–17

Julie rolls a 3 kg bowling ball down the bowling alley at a velocity of 7 m/s. Ken rolls a 5 kg bowling ball down the bowling alley at a velocity of 4 m/s. How does the momentum of the two bowling balls compare?

(A) Julie's ball has a momentum of 67 kg · m/s more than Ken's ball.

(B) Julie's ball has a momentum of 1 kg · m/s more than Ken's ball.

(C) Ken's ball has a momentum of 33 kg · m/s more than Julie's ball.

(D) Both balls have the same momentum.

Your Answer _____

Q–18

The Y chromosome carries fewer traits than the X chromosome. A male will transmit these traits to

(A) 100% of his female offspring

(B) 100% of his male offspring

(C) 50% of his female offspring

(D) 50% of his male offspring

Your Answer _____

Correct Answers

A–17

(B) Linear momentum of an object is defined as the product of its mass and the velocity:

$$p = mv$$

Julie's bowling ball has a mass of 3 kg and is moving at a velocity of 7 m/s; therefore, her ball has a momentum of 21 kg · m/s. Ken's bowling ball has a mass of 5 kg and is moving at a velocity of 4 m/s; therefore, his ball has a momentum of 20 kg · m/s.

A–18

(B) A male has both the X and Y chromosomes, while a female has two X chromosomes and no Y. Therefore, a male will pass all the traits on his Y chromosome to 100% of his male offspring. (D) is incorrect because a male will pass on all of the traits on his Y chromosome to all of his male offspring. (A) and (C) are incorrect because a female will receive the male's X chromosome, not his Y.

Questions

Q–19

What would be the cost of running a television with a resistance of 80.0 Ω for 24 hours if 120 volts is supplied? The electrical energy costs $0.085 per kW · h.

(A) $0.37

(B) $3.06

(C) $0.16

(D) $0.24

Your Answer _____

Correct Answers

A–19

(A)   In order to determine how much power the television is using, or how many watts, the amount of current used must first be determined. The amount of current used can be calculated using the resistance equation:

$$R = \Delta V/I \text{ or } I = \Delta V/R$$

Resistance = Potential Difference/Current, or Current = Potential Difference/Resistance

$$I = 120 \text{ V}/80.0 \text{ } \Omega = 1.5 \text{ A}$$

The electric power can then be calculated using the equation:

$$P = I\Delta V$$

Electric Power = Current × Potential Difference

$$P = 1.5 \text{ A} \times 120 \text{ V} = 180 \text{ W}$$

The cost of the electricity is in kilowatts, so the 180 watts needs to be converted to 0.180 kilowatts. The television runs for 24 hours; therefore, the cost is:

Cost = (0.180 kW)($0.085/kW · h)(24 h) = $0.37

Questions

Q–20

A cell can be thought of as an aqueous solution enclosed in a semi-permeable membrane. To keep cells from bursting or collapsing when patients receive fluids intravenously, what type of pressure must these fluids have to match that within cells?

(A) thermodynamic

(B) osmotic

(C) ionic

(D) exothermic

Your Answer _____

_____

Q–21

The following is a typical forest ecosystem food chain: grass → mouse → fox → owl. In this food chain, the fox's relationship to the mouse is best described as

(A) mutualism

(B) producer-consumer

(C) predator-prey

(D) parasitism

Your Answer _____

_____

Correct Answers

A–20

(B) It is important for intravenous fluids to have the same osmotic pressure as that within cells to keep cells from bursting or collapsing. Osmosis is the phenomenon of solvent flow through a semi-permeable membrane to equalize the solute concentrations on both sides of the membrane. Having equal osmotic pressure on both sides of the membrane stops osmotic flow. Thermodynamic relates to heat and other energy involved in chemical or physical processes. Ionic refers to charged particles. Exothermic involves a chemical reaction or physical change in which heat is released.

A–21

(C) Predator-prey is the correct answer. The fox acquires energy from the mouse in this food chain, so the fox is the predator and the mouse is the prey. (A) Mutualism refers to a type of symbiosis in which both organisms benefit. (B) Producer-consumer refers to the relationship between the grass and the mouse, where the grass is the producer of energy through photosynthesis and the mouse is the consumer as it eats the grass. (D) Parasitism refers to a type of symbiosis in which one organism benefits (the parasite) and the other organism is harmed (the host).

Questions

Q–22

What is the de Broglie wavelength of a 0.08 kg golf ball moving at 85 m/s?

(A) 6.80 m

(B) 9.41×10^4 m

(C) 9.75×10^{35} m

(D) 1.03×10^{34} m

Your Answer _____

_____

Q–23

Hornworts, liverworts, and mosses are examples of which type of plants?

(A) nonvascular

(B) gymnosperms

(C) angiosperms

(D) vascular

Your Answer _____

_____

Correct Answers

A–22

(C) French physicist Louis de Broglie proposed that all forms of matter may have both wave properties and particle properties. The wavelength of a photon was found to be equal to Planck's constant (h) divided by the photon's momentum (p). De Broglie speculated that this relationship would also hold true for matter waves:

$$\lambda = h/p = h/mv$$

de Broglie Wavelength

$$= \text{Planck's Constant/Momentum}$$

Planck's constant (h) = 6.63×10^{-34} J · s

$$\lambda = (6.63 \times 10^{-34} \text{ J} \cdot \text{s}) / (0.08 \text{ kg})(85 \text{ m/s})$$
$$\lambda = 9.75 \times 10^{-35} \text{ m}$$

A–23

(A) Nonvascular is the correct answer. All of these plants are nonvascular and transport water and nutrients from cell to cell through simple osmosis and diffusion. (D) Vascular plants have a xylem and phloem to transport water and nutrients. (B) Gymnosperms are a type of vascular plant characterized by "naked" seeds unprotected by fruit. (C) Angiosperms are a type of vascular plant characterized by seeds protected in fruit.

Questions

Q–24

As liquid water turns to water vapor, what happens to the entropy of this material?

(A) It increases.

(B) It decreases.

(C) It increases and decreases cyclically.

(D) It remains stable.

Your Answer _____

_____

Correct Answers

A–24

(A)   The entropy of liquid water increases as it becomes water vapor. This is true of any liquid that undergoes a phase change to become a gas, since the particles of a gas are less orderly than the particles of a liquid. As liquids become gases, entropy doesn't decrease, increase and decrease cyclically, or remain stable.

Questions

Q–25

A 2,300 kg car moving east at 11 m/s collides head-on with a 3,150 kg car moving west. The cars stick together and move as a unit after the collision at a velocity of 6.2 m/s to the west. What was the velocity of the 3,150 kg car prior to the collision?

(A)   2.70 m/s

(B)   17.20 m/s

(C)   6.36 m/s

(D)   18.76 m/s

Your Answer _____

_____

Correct Answers

A–25

(D) The conservation of momentum states that the total momentum will stay constant in an elastic collision. Momentum is calculated by an object's mass multiplied by its velocity. Therefore:

$$m_1 v_{1,i} + m_2 v_{2,i} = m_1 v_{1,f} + m_2 v_{2,f}$$

Since the cars were initially moving in opposite directions, one of the car's velocities will need to be expressed as a negative velocity in respect to the other car. In this case, the velocity to the east will be expressed as a positive velocity, and the velocity to the west will be expressed as a negative velocity. Also, because the cars stick together after the collision and move as one unit, the final momentums of both cars can be combined into one expression.

$$(2{,}300 \text{ kg})(11 \text{ m/s}) + (3{,}150 \text{ kg})(v_{2,i})$$
$$= (2{,}300 \text{ kg} + 3{,}150 \text{ kg})(-6.2 \text{ m/s})$$
$$25{,}300 \text{ kg} \cdot \text{m/s} + (3{,}150 \text{ kg})(v_{2,i})$$
$$= -33{,}790 \text{ kg} \cdot \text{m/s}$$
$$(3{,}150 \text{ kg})(v_{2,i})$$
$$= -59{,}090 \text{ kg} \cdot \text{m/s}$$
$$v_{2,i} = -18.76 \text{ m/s}$$

The negative velocity would indicate that the car was initially moving to the west.

Questions

Q–26

The roots of many clover plants produce structures that are filled with bacteria. The clover plants provide food and shelter for the bacteria, while the bacteria produce a nutrient that is used by the plants. As a result, clover plants that have these structures on their roots grow at a faster rate and are healthier than clover plants that do not have the structures. What type of relationship exists between the clover plants that have these structures on their roots and the bacteria in the structures?

(A) mutualism

(B) parasitism

(C) predator-prey

(D) commensalism

Your Answer _____

_____

Correct Answers

A–26

(A)   Mutualism is the correct answer. Symbiosis is when two organisms live closely together and one organism benefits. Mutualism is a type of symbiosis in which both organisms benefit. Since both the bacteria and the clover plants benefit, this symbiotic relationship is classified as mutualism. (B) Parasitism is a type of symbiosis in which one organism benefits and the other is harmed. (C) Predator-prey is a relationship in which one organism eats another and is not symbiotic. (D) Commensalism is a type of symbiosis in which one organism benefits and the other is neither hurt nor harmed.

Questions

Q–27

A 0.1 kg metal bolt is heated to a temperature of 85°C. It is then dropped into a beaker containing 0.3 kg of water with an unknown initial temperature. The bolt and the water then reach a final temperature of 27°C. If the metal has a specific heat capacity of 876 J/kg · °C, and water has a specific heat capacity of 4,186 J/kg · °C, what is the initial temperature of the water?

(A) 4°C

(B) 23°C

(C) 8°C

(D) 19°C

Your Answer _____

_____

Correct Answers

(B) Each substance has a unique value for the energy required to change the temperature of 1 kg of the substance by 1°C. This value is known as the substance's specific heat capacity. When the hot metal bolt is dropped into the cooler water, energy is released from the bolt and absorbed by the water until equilibrium is reached. This energy equilibrium can be expressed as:

$$c_{p,w} m_w \Delta T_w = c_{p,m} m_m \Delta T_m$$

where c_p = specific heat capacity, m = mass, and ΔT = change in temperature.

$(4{,}186 \text{ J/kg} \cdot °\text{C })(0.3 \text{ kg})(\Delta T_w)$
$\qquad = (876 \text{ J/kg} \cdot °\text{C})(0.1 \text{ kg})(85°\text{C} - 27°\text{C})$
$(1{,}255.8 \text{ J/°C})(\Delta T_w)$
$\qquad = 5{,}080.8 \text{ J}$
$\Delta T_w = 4°\text{C}$

Since this represents the change in temperature, the initial temperature was 23°C.

Questions

Q–28

A person with excess stomach acid, HCl, might take milk of magnesia, $Mg(OH)_2$, to relieve his or her discomfort. Which negative ions are formed in the chemical reaction that takes place?

(A) H^- and Mg^-

(B) Cl^- and OH^-

(C) H^- and Mg^{2-}

(D) Cl^- and OH^{2-}

Your Answer _____

_____

Q–29

Which of the following exerts the most pressure while resting on a floor?

(A) a 50-pound box with 3-foot sides

(B) a 40-pound box with 2-foot sides

(C) a 45-pound cylinder with a base radius of 1.5 feet

(D) a 10-pound cylinder with a base radius of 0.5 feet

Your Answer _____

_____

Correct Answers

A–28

(B) The negative ions that are formed when HCl reacts with $Mg(OH)_2$ are Cl^- and OH^-. H and Mg form positive ions, H^+ and Mg^{2+}.

A–29

(D) Pressure is a measure of how much force is applied over a given area.

$$P = F/A$$
Pressure = Force/Area

In answer choice (A), the 50-pound box covers an area of 9 square feet (3 ft × 3 ft). This box exerts a pressure on the floor of 5.55 lbs/ft². In answer choice (B), the 40-pound box covers an area of 4 square feet (2 ft × 2 ft). This box exerts a pressure on the floor of 10 lbs/ft². In answer choice (C), the 45-pound cylinder covers an area of 7.07 square feet ($\pi \times 1.5^2$). This cylinder exerts a pressure on the floor of 6.36 lbs/ft². In answer choice (D), the 10-pound cylinder covers an area of 0.785 square feet ($\pi \times 0.5^2$). This cylinder exerts a pressure on the floor of 12.74 lbs/ft². So despite the fact that this cylinder weighs considerably less than the other answer choices, it exerts the most pressure on the floor due to its small area.

Questions

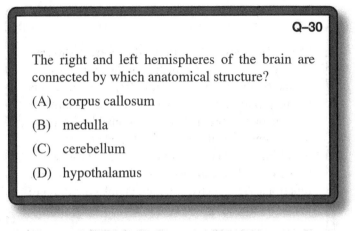

Q–30

The right and left hemispheres of the brain are connected by which anatomical structure?

(A)   corpus callosum

(B)   medulla

(C)   cerebellum

(D)   hypothalamus

Your Answer _____

_____

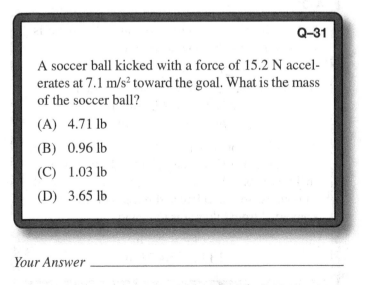

Q–31

A soccer ball kicked with a force of 15.2 N accelerates at 7.1 m/s² toward the goal. What is the mass of the soccer ball?

(A)   4.71 lb

(B)   0.96 lb

(C)   1.03 lb

(D)   3.65 lb

Your Answer _____

_____

Correct Answers

A–30

(A) Corpus callosum is the correct answer. The right and left hemispheres of the brain are connected by the corpus callosum. (B) The medulla is the respiratory, cardiac, vomiting, and vasomotor section of the brain that is responsible for autonomic functions like heart rate, blood pressure, and breathing. (C) The cerebellum is the largest part of the brain and is responsible for sensory and motor functions. (D) The hypothalamus links the brain to the endocrine system through the pituitary gland.

A–31

(A) Newton's second law states that force is proportional to mass and acceleration:

$$\Sigma F = ma$$

$$\text{Net External Force} = \text{Mass} \times \text{Acceleration}$$

$$15.2 \text{ N} = m \times (7.1 \text{ m/s}^2)$$

$$m = (15.2 \text{ N})/(7.1 \text{ m/s}^2) = 2.14 \text{ kg}$$

The weight component of the newton unit is in kilograms; therefore, the calculated mass is also in kilograms. The answer choices are expressed in pounds, so our calculated mass will need to be converted from kilograms to pounds.

$$1 \text{ kg} = 2.2 \text{ lb}$$

$$2.14 \text{ kg} = 4.71 \text{ lb}$$

Questions

Q–32

The temperature range of one northwestern state varies from 97°F in the summer to −15°F in the winter. What is this temperature range on the Kelvin scale?

(A) 36.1 K to −26.1 K

(B) 309.1 K to 246.9 K

(C) 206.6 K to 5.0 K

(D) 370.0 K to 258.0 K

Your Answer _____

Q–33

In oxygen gas, where each atom of oxygen exerts an equal attraction to the pair's shared electrons, what is the oxygen atoms' oxidation state?

(A) zero

(B) one

(C) two

(D) three

Your Answer _____

Correct Answers

A–32

(B) The most widely used temperature scales are the Fahrenheit, Celsius, and Kelvin scales. The Fahrenheit scale is most commonly used in the United States. The Kelvin scale, also known as the absolute scale, is always positive. The temperature of 0 K is often referred to as absolute zero.

In order to convert from the Fahrenheit scale to the Kelvin scale, the following formula can be used:

$$K = [(°F - 32) \times \tfrac{5}{9}] + 273$$

To convert 97°F to K:

$$K = [(97°F - 32) \times \tfrac{5}{9}] + 273$$
$$K = 309.1 \text{ K}$$

To convert $-15°F$ to K:

$$K = [(-15°F - 32) \times \tfrac{5}{9}] + 273$$
$$K = 246.9°K$$

A–33

(A) In oxygen gas, and other compounds where electrons are shared equally among atoms, the individual atoms have a zero oxidation state. If electrons were shared unequally, the atoms might have higher positive or negative oxidation states.

Questions

Q–34

Polar bears have a layer of fat to insulate them from cold and thick, water-resistant fur that serves as camouflage. Which term best describes these characteristics?

(A) adaptation

(B) natural selection

(C) alteration

(D) mutation

Your Answer _____

_____

Q–35

Visible light, radio waves, and X-rays are all types of electromagnetic waves. These types of electromagnetic waves are distinguished by their different:

(A) temperatures

(B) amplitudes

(C) wavelengths

(D) intensities

Your Answer _____

_____

Correct Answers

A–34

(A) Adaptation is the correct answer. Adaptations are traits that improve an organism's chance of survival and eventual reproduction. (B) Natural selection is the basic explanation for evolution, whereby the most fit organisms are more likely to survive and reproduce more, influencing the next generation by passing on more of their traits to the population. (C) Alteration has no biological meaning in this context. (D) Mutations are changes in DNA that lead to different or incorrect gene expression.

A–35

(C) Electromagnetic waves are distinguished by their different frequencies and wavelengths. Visible light has a wavelength range of 700 nm for red to 400 nm for violet. Radio waves have relatively long wavelengths of more than 30 cm. X-rays, on the other hand, have short wavelengths, ranging from 60 nm to 10^{-4} nm.

Questions

Q–36

Methane, the principal component of natural gas, has the chemical formula CH_4. Why is it considered a saturated hydrocarbon?

(A) It dissolves easily in water.

(B) It readily soaks through fabric.

(C) Its scent quickly fills rooms.

(D) Its carbon atoms are bound to the maximum number of hydrogen atoms.

Your Answer _____

_____

Q–37

When one base of DNA is accidentally deleted during transcription, the resulting amino acid sequence will be greatly affected, resulting in a major mutation. Which type of point mutation does this scenario describe?

(A) chain termination

(B) frame shift

(C) neutral

(D) translocation

Your Answer _____

_____

Correct Answers

A–36

(D) Methane is considered a saturated hydrocarbon because all of its carbon atoms are bound to the maximum number of hydrogen atoms. Saturated hydrocarbons are not defined by their ability to dissolve in water, soak through fabric, or spread their scent through rooms. Other saturated hydrocarbons include paraffin and octane.

A–37

(B) Frame shift is the correct answer. Consider the analogy "THE FAT CAT ATE THE RAT." Deleting the F in FAT makes the sentence read, "THE ATC ATA TET HER AT." Just as the sentence no longer makes sense, when one base is deleted from a DNA sequence, the entire reading frame shifts. Codons become nonsense downstream from the point of mutation. (A) A chain termination mutation occurs when one of the bases of a stop codon is altered such that transcription of DNA does not stop at the appropriate place. (C) There is some duplication of codons when mRNA is transcribed to amino acids. If one of the DNA bases changes, but the corresponding amino acid does not, the result is a neutral mutation. (D) A translocation mutation is a chromosomal mutation, not a point mutation.

Questions

Q-38

A skateboarder is traveling at 5 m/s. During a 13-second period, the skateboarder slows down at a constant acceleration to a speed of 1 m/s. How far does the skateboarder travel during this 13-second time period?

(A) 52 meters

(B) 78 meters

(C) 26 meters

(D) 39 meters

Your Answer _____

Q-39

According to Charles's law, what will a blown-up balloon do if you take it from a warm room to outside on a chilly day?

(A) grow

(B) shrink

(C) pop

(D) stay stable

Your Answer _____

Correct Answers

A–38

(D) For motion with a constant acceleration, the displacement with respect to time can be solved by the following relationship:

$$\Delta x = \tfrac{1}{2}(v_i + v_f)\Delta t$$

Displacement =
$\tfrac{1}{2}$(Initial Velocity + Final Velocity)(Time Interval)

$$\Delta x = \tfrac{1}{2}\,(5 \text{ m/s} + 1 \text{ m/s})(13 \text{ s})$$

$$\Delta x = 39 \text{ meters}$$

A–39

(B) According to Charles's law, a blown-up balloon will shrink when you take it from a warm room to outside on a chilly day. Charles's law states that the volume occupied by a sample of gas at a constant pressure is directly proportional to the absolute temperature. As such, when temperature decreases, the volume of gas will also decrease. Conversely, as temperature increases, the volume of gas will increase.

Questions

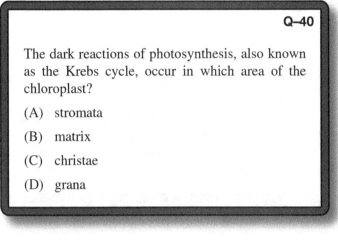

Q–40

The dark reactions of photosynthesis, also known as the Krebs cycle, occur in which area of the chloroplast?

(A) stromata

(B) matrix

(C) christae

(D) grana

Your Answer _____

_____

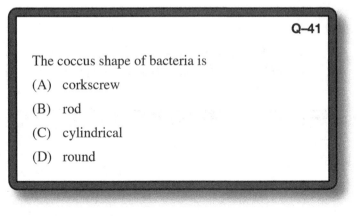

Q–41

The coccus shape of bacteria is

(A) corkscrew

(B) rod

(C) cylindrical

(D) round

Your Answer _____

_____

Correct Answers

A–40

(A) Stromata is the correct answer. The dark reactions of photosynthesis occur in the stromata of the chloroplast. (D) The light reactions of photosynthesis occur in the grana of the chloroplast. (B) The matrix of the mitochondria is the site of the Calvin cycle in cellular respiration, and (C) the christae of the mitochondria are the site of chemiosmotic phosphorylation in cellular respiration.

A–41

(D) Round is the correct answer. Coccus refers to round or spherical bacterial. The other answers are incorrect.

Questions

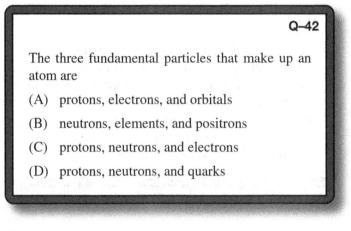

Q–42

The three fundamental particles that make up an atom are

(A) protons, electrons, and orbitals

(B) neutrons, elements, and positrons

(C) protons, neutrons, and electrons

(D) protons, neutrons, and quarks

Your Answer _____

_____

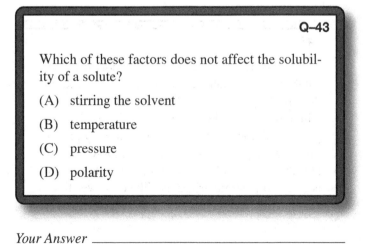

Q–43

Which of these factors does not affect the solubility of a solute?

(A) stirring the solvent

(B) temperature

(C) pressure

(D) polarity

Your Answer _____

_____

Correct Answers

A-42

(C) Protons, neutrons, and electrons are the fundamental particles that make up an atom. Orbitals are locations that electrons occupy outside an atom's nucleus. Positrons are similar to electrons, but have a positive charge instead of a negative charge as electrons do. Quarks are the basic building blocks of protons and neutrons.

A-43

(A) Stirring the solvent does not affect the solubility of a solute, though it may speed the dissolving process. Solubility typically increases with temperature. Pressure affects the solubility of gases, with the solubility of a gas directly proportional to the pressure of the gas. In most cases, solutes dissolve in solvents with similar polarity. This is commonly summarized as "like dissolves like."

Questions

Q–44

A car with an initial speed of 5.5 m/s accelerates at a uniform rate of 2.3 m/s². How fast is the car traveling after 8 seconds?

(A)   15.8 m/s

(B)   46.3 m/s

(C)   23.9 m/s

(D)   18.4 m/s

Your Answer _____

_____

Q–45

The function of the ribosome is

(A)   translocation

(B)   transcription

(C)   replication

(D)   translation

Your Answer _____

_____

Correct Answers

A–44

(C) The final velocity of the car is dependent on the initial velocity, the rate of acceleration, and the time interval. The relationship is as follows:

$$v_f = v_i + a\Delta t$$

final velocity = initial velocity
+ (acceleration × time interval)

The car had an initial velocity of 5.5 m/s. Its acceleration was 2.3 m/s² for a time period of 8 seconds:

$$
\begin{aligned}
v_f &= 5.5 \text{ m/s} + (2.3 \text{ m/s}^2 \times 8 \text{ s}) \\
&= 5.5 \text{ m/s} + 18.4 \text{ m/s} \\
&= 23.9 \text{ m/s}
\end{aligned}
$$

A–45

(D) The ribosome is the site of translation, where mRNA is paired with tRNA as amino acids are linked together into a protein. Translocation is an example of a chromosomal mutation in which part of a chromosome detaches and reattaches to another chromosome. Transcription occurs in the nucleus where the base sequence of a particular gene is recoded by enzymes from DNA into mRNA. Replication occurs in the nucleus during the S phase of the cell cycle. During this process, DNA unzips and enzymes produce two identical copies of the original DNA.

Questions

Q–46

How much power is required to carry a 42-newton box a vertical distance of 21 meters if the work on the package is accomplished in 38 seconds?

(A) 23.2 W

(B) 76.0 W

(C) 1.7 W

(D) 0.6 W

Your Answer _____

Q–47

In fruit flies, the gene for green eyes (G) is dominant to the gene for white eyes (g). If the offspring is 76 fruit flies with green eyes and 22 fruit flies with white eyes, what are the most likely genotypes of the parents?

(A) GG and GG

(B) Gg and Gg

(C) Gg and gg

(D) gg and gg

Your Answer _____

Correct Answers

(A) Power is defined as the rate at which work is done.

$$P = W/\Delta t$$

Work is defined as the magnitude of the force multiplied by the distance the force is moved.

$$W = Fd$$
$$P = Fd/\Delta t$$
$$P = (42 \text{ N})(21 \text{ m})/(38 \text{ s})$$
$$P = 23.2 \text{ W}$$

(B) Gg and Gg is the correct answer. The ratio of fruit flies most closely corresponds to a 3:1 ratio. Solving Punnett squares for each option only yields a 3:1 ratio for (B) Gg and Gg (75% of offspring are predicted to have at least one dominant allele and 25% are predicted to be recessive). None of the other Punnett squares produce this ratio; (A) GG and GG predict 100% dominant, (C) Gg and gg predict 50% dominant and 50% recessive, and (D) gg and gg predict 100% recessive.

Questions

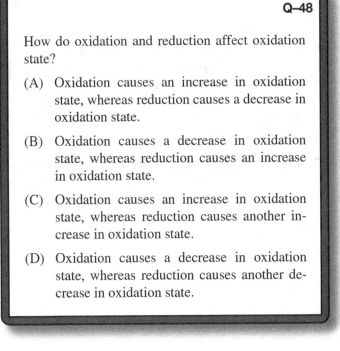

How do oxidation and reduction affect oxidation state?

(A) Oxidation causes an increase in oxidation state, whereas reduction causes a decrease in oxidation state.

(B) Oxidation causes a decrease in oxidation state, whereas reduction causes an increase in oxidation state.

(C) Oxidation causes an increase in oxidation state, whereas reduction causes another increase in oxidation state.

(D) Oxidation causes a decrease in oxidation state, whereas reduction causes another decrease in oxidation state.

Your Answer _____

_____

Correct Answers

A–48

(A) Oxidation involves an increase in oxidation state; reduction involves a decrease in oxidation state. This is usually thought of as atoms, ions, or molecules losing electrons when they are oxidized and gaining electrons when they are reduced. Oxidation does not involve decreasing oxidation state, nor does reduction involve increasing it.

Questions

Q–49

While on Earth, an astronaut weighs 180 pounds and has a mass of about 18 pounds. While on the moon, the astronaut weighs about 30 pounds. What is the astronaut's mass on the moon?

(A) 3 pounds

(B) 30 pounds

(C) 180 pounds

(D) 18 pounds

Your Answer _____

Q–50

A 9 V battery is connected to a light bulb that has a current running through it of 2.14 A. What is the resistance in the light bulb?

(A) 19.26 Ω

(B) 0.24 Ω

(C) 4.2 Ω

(D) 9.63 Ω

Your Answer _____

Correct Answers

A–49

(D) The weight of an object depends on the force of gravity acting on it. Because there is less gravity on the moon, the weight of the astronaut will be less on the moon than it is on Earth. However, mass is a measure of the amount of matter contained in the object and is not dependent on the force of gravity. Therefore, the astronaut's mass is the same on the moon as it is on Earth.

A–50

(C) Most materials can be classified as either conductors or insulators. Some conductors allow electric charges to move through them more easily than others. The opposition to the motion of the electric charge through a conductor is known as the conductor's resistance. The resistance of a material can be calculated as the ratio of the potential difference (or voltage) to current:

$$R = \Delta V/I$$
Resistance = Potential Difference/Current

Therefore, if a 9 V battery is used and a current of 2.14 A is seen, the resistance of the bulb would be:

$$R = 9 \text{ V}/2.14 \text{ A}$$
$$R = 4.2 \ \Omega$$

Questions

Q–51

A 12.0 V battery is connected to five resistors, which are connected together in parallel. The resistance of each resistor, in order from the battery to the end, is 3 Ω, 4 Ω, 5 Ω, 6 Ω, and 7 Ω. What is the total current in the circuit?

(A) 0.48 A

(B) 13.09 A

(C) 2.08 A

(D) 0.08 A

Q–52

The stage of mitosis in which DNA is condensed into chromosomes, aligned at the equatorial plane, and attached to spindle fibers from the centrioles is best described as

(A) metaphase

(B) telophase

(C) anaphase

(D) interphase

Your Answer _____

_____

Correct Answers

A–51

(B) When resistors are connected in parallel, the equivalent total resistance of the circuit can be calculated using a reciprocal relationship:

$$1/R_{eq} = 1/R_1 + 1/R_2 + 1/R_3 + \ldots$$

Therefore, the equivalent total resistance of the given circuit is:

$$1/R_{eq} = 1/3\ \Omega + 1/4\ \Omega + 1/5\ \Omega + 1/6\ \Omega + 1/7\ \Omega$$
$$1/R_{eq} = 1.09/1\ \Omega$$
$$R_{eq} = 0.917\ \Omega$$

The total current in the circuit is equivalent to the potential difference divided by the equivalent resistance:

$$I = \Delta V/R_{eq}$$
$$I = 12\ \text{V}/0.917\ \Omega$$
$$I = 13.09\ \text{A}$$

A–52

(A) Metaphase is the correct answer. During interphase, DNA exists as chromatin. During anaphase, centrioles pull apart chromosomes into chromatids. During telophase, the chromatids begin to relax into chromatin and the nucleus begins to reform in each daughter cell, just prior to cytokinesis.

Questions

Q-53

Varieties of the same element can have the same number of protons but different numbers of neutrons. What are these varieties called?

(A) anions

(B) isolates

(C) isotopes

(D) valences

Your Answer _____

_____

Q-54

You might be able to tell that a chemical reaction has taken place between two compounds by noticing

(A) light

(B) heat

(C) a color change

(D) all of the above

Your Answer _____

_____

Correct Answers

A-53

(C)   Isotopes are varieties of the same element that have the same number of protons but different numbers of neutrons. Anions are negatively charged atoms or groups of atoms. Isolates are elements or compounds that have been purified from a mixture. Valence refers to the electrons in the outer shell of an atom.

A-54

(D)   A chemical reaction is a change in which two or more kinds of matter are transformed into a new kind of matter or several new kinds of matter. It is typically accompanied by detectable changes, including light, heat, or a color change.

Questions

Q–55

Betty accidentally runs out of gas in her car one morning on her way to the hospital. She sees a gas station on the next block and decides to attempt to push her car to the station. Betty exerts a force of 200 newtons on the car. She tries pushing the car for 20 minutes, to the point of sweating and exhaustion, but is unable to move the car at all. How much work did Betty do on the car?

(A) 0 joules

(B) 66.67 joules

(C) 200 joules

(D) 4,000 joules

Your Answer _____

_____

Correct Answers

A–55

(A) Despite the fact that Betty exerted a force on the car, and pushed to the point of exhaustion, no work was done on the car. In order for work to be done, the car would have had to move. The amount of work done on an object is defined as the amount of force applied to the object times the magnitude of the displacement, or movement, of the object:

$$\text{work} = \text{force} \times \text{distance}$$

So even though Betty applied as much force to the car as she was able to, no work was done on the car because the car did not move.

Questions

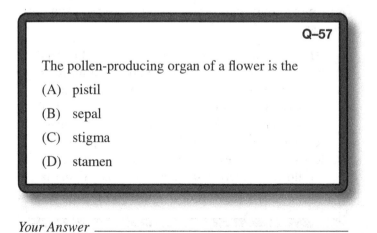

Q–56

A 4.0 kg ball rolling to the right at 7 m/s has an elastic head-on collision with a 6 kg ball that is initially at rest. After the collision, the 4.0 kg ball continues to roll to the right at a velocity of 3 m/s. How fast is the 6 kg ball rolling after the collision?

(A)   2 m/s

(B)   2.67 m/s

(C)   4.67 m/s

(D)   16 m/s

Your Answer _____

Q–57

The pollen-producing organ of a flower is the

(A)   pistil

(B)   sepal

(C)   stigma

(D)   stamen

Your Answer _____

Correct Answers

A-56

(B) The conservation of momentum states that the total initial momentum will equal the total final momentum. In other words, the total momentum of the 4 kg ball and the 6 kg ball prior to the collision will equal the total momentum of the two balls after the collision.

$$m_1 v_{1,i} + m_2 v_{2,i} = m_1 v_{1,f} + m_2 v_{2,f}$$
$$(4 \text{ kg})(7 \text{ m/s}) + (6 \text{ kg})(0 \text{ m/s})$$
$$= (4 \text{ kg})(3 \text{ m/s}) + (6 \text{ kg})(v_{2,f})$$
$$28 \text{ kg} \cdot \text{m/s} = 12 \text{ kg} \cdot \text{m/s} + (6 \text{ kg})(v_{2,f})$$
$$v_{2,f} = 2.67 \text{ m/s}$$

A-57

(D) Stamen is the correct answer. Flowers produce pollen through their stamen, the flower's male reproductive organ. Specifically, pollen is produced on the anther, the structure at the end of the stamen. (A) The pistil is the flower's female reproductive organ. (B) Sepals are green protective leaf-like structures that cover the flower petals and the flower's internal structure. (C) The stigma is the sticky end of the pistil and captures pollen.

Questions

Q–58

Although mitosis is commonly referred to as cell division, the cell itself truly becomes two separate cells through which process?

(A) telophase

(B) cytokinesis

(C) s phase

(D) transcription

Your Answer _____

_____

Q–59

The bonding capacity of an atom is determined by its number of

(A) protons

(B) neutrons

(C) electrons

(D) valence electrons

Your Answer _____

_____

Correct Answers

A–58

(B) Cytokinesis is the correct answer. Cytokinesis, or the pinching of the cell membrane, occurs at the end of telophase. After cytokinesis, two separate daughter cells exist. (A) During telophase, there are two nuclei, but they are contained within the same cell. (C) S phase is the name for mitosis (nuclear division) in the cellular cycle. (D) Transcription is the process of moving genetic information from DNA to mRNA.

A–59

(D) Valence electrons determine the bonding capacity of an atom. These electrons are completely transferred to other atoms in ionic bonds and shared between atoms in covalent bonds. Bonding capacity doesn't depend on protons, neutrons, or electrons other than valence electrons.

Questions

Q–60

The laws of thermodynamics control which way chemical reactions proceed. What can you predict about the direction of spontaneous chemical reactions based on thermodynamics?

(A) They will proceed in the direction that decreases energy.

(B) They will proceed in the direction that increases enthalpy.

(C) They will proceed in the direction that decreases entropy.

(D) They will proceed in the direction that increases entropy.

Your Answer _____

_____

Q–61

What is the wavelength of an FM radio signal if the number on the dial reads 92.3 MHz?

(A) 92.3 m

(B) 325 m

(C) 0.003 m

(D) 30.7 m

Your Answer _____

_____

Correct Answers

A–60

(D) Spontaneous chemical reactions will proceed in the direction that increases entropy, based on the second law of thermodynamics. They will not proceed in a direction that increases energy, since energy can neither be created nor destroyed, according to the first law of thermodynamics. Spontaneous chemical reactions also cannot proceed in a direction that increases enthalpy, or heat of a system, since heat is a form of energy and cannot be created or destroyed.

A–61

(B) All electromagnetic waves move at the speed of light. The relationship in an FM radio signal is given by the wave speed equation:

$$c = f\lambda$$
speed of light = frequency × wavelength

Therefore

$$\lambda = c/f$$
wavelength = speed of light/frequency

The speed of light (c) is approximately 3.00×10^8 m/s. A frequency of 92.3 MHz is equivalent to 9.23×10^5 Hz. Therefore

$$\lambda = (3.00 \times 10^8 \text{ m/s})/(9.23 \times 10^5 \text{ Hz})$$
$$\lambda = 325 \text{ m}$$

Questions

Q–62

All of the following about RNA are true EXCEPT

(A) RNA is single stranded

(B) RNA's nucleic acids include uracil instead of guanine

(C) RNA's sugar-phosphate backbone contains ribose

(D) RNA permeates the nuclear envelope

Your Answer _____

Q–63

In a certain species of moth, there are two phenotypes: white with brown spots and brown with white spots. What is the name of the theory that predicts that the brown moths with white spots will reproduce more and that future generations will have higher percentages of this phenotype represented in future generations in an environment where tree bark is predominantly brown?

(A) competition

(B) natural selection

(C) symbiosis

(D) theory of use and disuse

Your Answer _____

Correct Answers

A–62

(B) RNA contains uracil and guanine, in addition to adenine and cytosine. RNA contains uracil instead of thiamine. The other statements are true.

A–63

(B) Natural selection, also referred to as survival of the fittest, is the theory Charles Darwin developed that states that organisms that are more fit and that are best suited to their environment reproduce more and have a bigger impact on the next generation. Competition occurs between members of the same species as they fight for limited resources such as food. Symbiosis is when two organisms live closely together and at least one member benefits. The theory of use and disuse is derived from Lamarck's incorrect theory of evolution. In this theory, a giraffe's long neck elongates as it is used for eating leaves from the tops of tall trees.

Questions

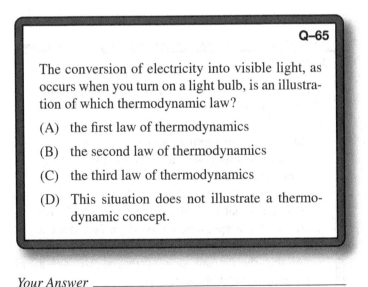

Q-64

Brandi lifts a 40 kg box 2 meters off the ground in 3 seconds. If she had taken 6 seconds to lift the box, the work done on the box would have been

(A)   twice as great

(B)   four times as great

(C)   the same

(D)   half as great

Your Answer _____

_____

Q-65

The conversion of electricity into visible light, as occurs when you turn on a light bulb, is an illustration of which thermodynamic law?

(A)   the first law of thermodynamics

(B)   the second law of thermodynamics

(C)   the third law of thermodynamics

(D)   This situation does not illustrate a thermo-dynamic concept.

Your Answer _____

Correct Answers

A–64

(C) Work is defined as the force applied to an object times the distance that the object is moved.

$$W = Fd$$
$$\text{Work} = \text{Force} \times \text{Distance}$$

Work is not dependent on time, so even though Brandi takes twice as long to lift the box, the amount of work that she does on the box remains the same.

A–65

(A) The conversion of electricity into visible light is an illustration of the first law of thermodynamics, which states that energy can change from one form to another, but cannot be created or destroyed. In this case, electrical energy is being converted into light energy. This situation is not an illustration of the second law of thermodynamics, which states that the entropy of a system always increases for a spontaneous process. Nor does it illustrate the third law of thermodynamics, which states that the entropy of a system approaches a minimum value at absolute zero.

Questions

Q–66

Which atomic symbol is based on the element's Latin name?

(A) Ds

(B) V

(C) Bi

(D) Hg

Your Answer _____

Q–67

The efficiency of a given pulley system is 82%. The pulleys are used to raise a mass to a certain height. What force is exerted on the system if a rope is pulled 19.0 m in order to raise a 64 kg mass a height of 3.5 m?

(A) 14.4 N

(B) 141.0 N

(C) 94.8 N

(D) 9.7 N

Your Answer _____

Correct Answers

A–66

(D) Hg is the symbol for mercury, which is based on the Latin word *hydragyrum*. Ds is the symbol for darmstadtium. V is the symbol for vanadium. Bi is the symbol for bismuth.

A–67

(B) The efficiency of a simple machine, such as a pulley system, is a measure of how much of the input energy is lost compared with how much energy is used to perform work on an object. In most cases, the lost energy is dissipated as friction.

$$eff = W_{out}/W_{in}$$
Efficiency = Work Out/Work In

Work is defined as force applied to an object multiplied by the distance the object is moved.

$$W = Fd$$
Work = Force × Distance

To calculate the force of the 64 kg mass, the effect of gravity must be taken into account.

$$W_{out} = (64 \text{ kg})(9.81 \text{ m/s}^2)(3.5 \text{ m}) = 2{,}197.4 \text{ J}$$

Efficiency: $0.82 = 2{,}197.4 \text{ J}/W_{in}$

$$W_{in} = 2{,}197.4 \text{ J}/0.82$$
$$W_{in} = 2{,}679.8 \text{ J}$$
$$F_{in} (19 \text{ m}) = 2{,}679.8 \text{ J}$$
$$F_{in} = 141.0 \text{ N}$$

Questions

Q–68

In the following gene, represented by the DNA sequence TCT GCA ACG, first T is changed to an A in a point mutation. The most likely cause for the mutation is

(A) butane gas

(B) acid rain

(C) ultraviolet light

(D) heavy metals

Your Answer _____

_____

Correct Answers

A–68

(C) Ultraviolet light is the correct answer. UV radiation can cause point mutations in DNA such as the one described above. Although toxic, neither (A) butane gas nor (C) heavy metals have known pathophysiologies that cause point mutations. Similarly, (B) acid rain is neither toxic nor known to cause point mutations.

Questions

Q–69

To study cellular respiration, a science student places yeast in a zipper bag with grapes. The grapes are gently crushed, the contents are mixed, and the air is removed from the bag with a straw before being sealed. Then, the bag is left overnight. The following morning, the bag is full of air. Which of the following statements correctly explains the experiment?

(A) As the yeast break down the sugar in the grapes, they produce oxygen as a by-product of cellular respiration.

(B) As the yeast break down the sugar in the grapes, they produce carbon dioxide as a by-product of cellular respiration.

(C) The yeast cells multiply rapidly through mitosis, causing the bag to expand.

(D) The yeast cells multiply rapidly through meiosis, causing the bag to expand.

Your Answer _____

Correct Answers

A–69

(B)   is the correct answer. The process occurring is cellular respiration (glucose + oxygen → chemical energy + carbon dioxide + water). The yeast are breaking down the glucose in the grapes to produce chemical energy; the gas present is carbon dioxide. (B) is incorrect since cellular respiration does not produce oxygen as a by-product. Neither (C) nor (D) is correct because mitosis and meiosis are processes of cell division that do not produce gas.

Questions

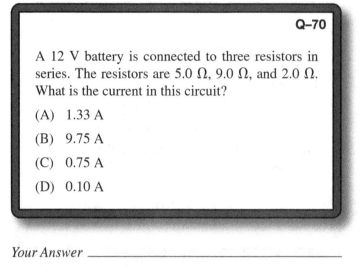

Q–70

A 12 V battery is connected to three resistors in series. The resistors are 5.0 Ω, 9.0 Ω, and 2.0 Ω. What is the current in this circuit?

(A) 1.33 A

(B) 9.75 A

(C) 0.75 A

(D) 0.10 A

Your Answer _____

_____

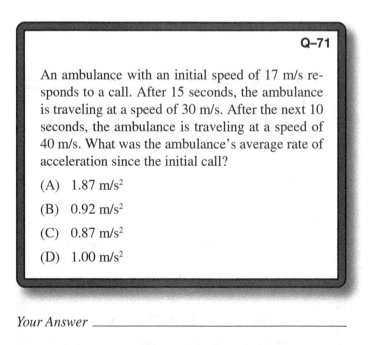

Q–71

An ambulance with an initial speed of 17 m/s responds to a call. After 15 seconds, the ambulance is traveling at a speed of 30 m/s. After the next 10 seconds, the ambulance is traveling at a speed of 40 m/s. What was the ambulance's average rate of acceleration since the initial call?

(A) 1.87 m/s^2

(B) 0.92 m/s^2

(C) 0.87 m/s^2

(D) 1.00 m/s^2

Your Answer _____

_____

Correct Answers

A–70

(C) The equivalent resistance of resistors connected in series equals the sum of the individual resistances.

$$R_{eq} = 5.0 \ \Omega + 9.0 \ \Omega + 2.0 \ \Omega = 16.0 \ \Omega$$

The current in a circuit can be calculated by dividing the potential difference by the equivalent resistance:

$$I = \Delta V/R_{eq}$$
$$I = 12 \ V/16 \ \Omega$$
$$I = 0.75 \ A$$

A–71

(B) The average rate of acceleration of the ambulance is dependent on the initial velocity, the final velocity, and the time interval. The relationship is as follows:

$$v_f = v_i + a\Delta t$$
or
$$a = (v_f - v_i)/\Delta t$$

The ambulance's initial speed was 17 m/s. The final speed was 40 m/s. It took the ambulance a total of 25 seconds to reach this speed. Therefore, the average rate of acceleration is:

$$a = (40 \ m/s - 17 \ m/s)/(25 \ s) = 0.92 \ m/s^2$$

Questions

Q-72

Absolute zero, or 0 kelvin, is considered the lowest temperature theoretically possible. Scientists have been able to attain temperatures close to absolute zero in the lab, but haven't yet been able to reach this very low temperature. At absolute zero, what do scientists theorize happens to the motion of particles?

(A) The motion dramatically increases.

(B) The motion dramatically slows.

(C) The motion stops.

(D) The motion of particles does not change once they reach absolute zero.

Your Answer _____

Q-73

What is a substance or combination of substances capable of neutralizing limited quantities of either an acid or a base that are added to it without significantly altering its pH value?

(A) neutral solution

(B) hydroxide ion

(C) hydronium ion

(D) buffer

Your Answer _____

Correct Answers

A–72

(C) The motion of particles is theorized to stop at absolute zero. This theory is in accordance with the third law of thermodynamics, which states that entropy decreases as the energy or temperature of a system decreases. At absolute zero, the energy of the system is at its theoretically lowest value. Consequently, the motion of particles doesn't increase, slow, or show no change at absolute zero.

A–73

(D) A buffer is a substance or combination of substances capable of neutralizing limited quantities of either an acid or a base that are added to it without significantly altering its pH value. A neutral solution is a substance with a pH of 7. A hydroxide ion, or OH^-, increases in concentration in an aqueous solution when a base is dissolved. A hydronium ion, or H_3O^+, increases in concentration in an aqueous solution when an acid is dissolved.

Questions

Q-74

While sitting at a stoplight, you hear the sound of an ambulance siren. The pitch of the siren continues to increase. Even though you can't yet see the ambulance, you know the ambulance is

(A) moving toward you

(B) moving away from you

(C) sitting still

(D) moving in an undetermined direction

Your Answer _____

Q-75

An ambulance is sounding its siren as it is moving east at 40 m/s. A car in front of the ambulance is moving east at 35 m/s. A pickup truck behind the ambulance is moving east at 30 m/s. A motorcyclist farther ahead of the car is sitting still along the side of the road. Which observer hears the ambulance siren at the highest pitch?

(A) the driver of the car

(B) the driver of the pickup truck

(C) the motorcyclist

(D) They all hear the same pitch.

Your Answer _____

Correct Answers

A–74

(A) If the source of the sound is moving toward the observer, the observer will hear the sound at an increasing pitch. Conversely, if the source of the sound is moving away from the observer, the observer will hear the sound at a decreasing pitch. This apparent change in the frequency of sound, due to the movement of either the source of the sound or the observer, is called the Doppler effect.

A–75

(C) The frequency of a sound wave determines its pitch. Although the frequency of the siren remains constant, because the ambulance is moving, the wave front reaches an observer in front of the ambulance more often than it would if the ambulance was stationary. Therefore, the frequency heard by the observers in front of the moving ambulance is greater than the source frequency. This shift in frequency is known as the Doppler effect. Since the motorcyclist is sitting still, the sound wave source is moving toward the motorcyclist at a velocity of 40 m/s. The car is also in front of the ambulance and would thus experience an increase in the pitch of the sound. However, because the car is also moving east at 35 m/s, the relative velocity increase of the ambulance is only 5 m/s. Thus, the increase in frequency due to the Doppler effect will not be as pronounced as the increase in frequency observed by the stationary motorcyclist.

Questions

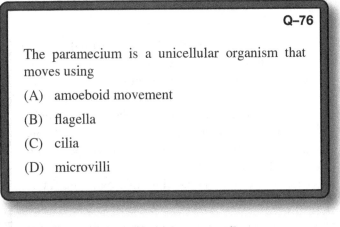

Q–76

The paramecium is a unicellular organism that moves using

(A) amoeboid movement

(B) flagella

(C) cilia

(D) microvilli

Your Answer _____

_____

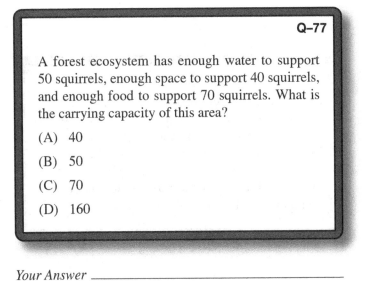

Q–77

A forest ecosystem has enough water to support 50 squirrels, enough space to support 40 squirrels, and enough food to support 70 squirrels. What is the carrying capacity of this area?

(A) 40

(B) 50

(C) 70

(D) 160

Your Answer _____

_____

Correct Answers

A–76

(C) The paramecium moves by rhythmically beating thousands of tiny hair-like cilia on the outside of its body. Amoeboid movement describes a snail-like movement in which arm-like cellular protrusions of the cell membrane assist the amoeba and other sarcodines in moving. The flagella are the tail-like protrusions that whip to propel flagellates like the volvox. Although similar to cilia and capable of rhythmic beating, microvilli are found in multicellular organisms.

A–77

(A) The correct answer is 40. Since there is only enough space to support 40 squirrels, 40 is the carrying capacity. The carry capacity of an ecosystem is equal to the lowest limiting factor. The other limiting factors, (B) 50 and (C) 70, surpass the lowest limiting factor. (D) 160 does not represent a limiting factor for this ecosystem.

Questions

Q–78

Suppose you start with 2.00×10^{-4} grams of a pure radioactive substance. You determine that 6.0 hours later, only 2.5×10^{-5} grams of the substance is left undecayed. What is the half-life of the substance?

(A) 2 hours

(B) 4 hours

(C) 6 hours

(D) 8 hours

Your Answer _____

_____

Correct Answers

A–78

(A)   The half-life of a radioactive substance is the time it takes for half of a given number of radioactive nuclei to decay. Beginning with 2.00×10^{-4} grams of a pure radioactive substance, after one half-life, 1.00×10^{-4} grams of the substance will still be radioactive. After another half-life, 5.00×10^{-5} grams of the substance will be radioactive. After a third half-life, 2.5×10^{-5} grams of the substance will still be radioactive. The three half-life time periods took place over a 6-hour period; therefore, the half-life of the substance is 2 hours.

Questions

Q–79

Anna has a mass of 30 kg. Starting from rest, she zooms down a frictionless slide from an initial height of 4.00 m above the ground. What is Anna's speed at the bottom of the slide?

(A)   not enough information given to calculate

(B)   120 m/s

(C)   78.48 m/s

(D)   8.86 m/s

Your Answer _____

_____

Correct Answers

A–79

(D) Since the slide is frictionless, mechanical energy is conserved. Therefore, the total energy (potential energy + kinetic energy) at the top of the slide is equal to the total energy at the bottom of the slide:

$$PE_i + KE_i = PE_f + KE_f$$

Because Anna starts from rest, the initial kinetic energy (KE_i) is zero. Likewise, because she is at a height of zero at the bottom of the slide, the final potential energy (PE_f) is also zero. The initial potential energy (PE_i) is calculated using Anna's mass, Earth's gravitational acceleration, and the height of the slide:

$$PE_i = mgh_i = (30 \text{ kg})(9.81 \text{ m/s}^2)(4 \text{ m}) = 1{,}177.2 \text{ J}$$

The final kinetic energy (KE_f) is calculated using Anna's mass and the velocity:

$$KE_f = \tfrac{1}{2} mv^2 = \tfrac{1}{2}(30 \text{ kg})(v^2)$$

Using the conservation of energy:

$$PE_i + KE_i = PE_f + KE_f$$
$$1{,}177.2 \text{ J} + 0 \text{ J} = 0 \text{ J} + \tfrac{1}{2}(30 \text{ kg})(v^2)$$
$$v^2 = 78.48 \text{ m}^2/\text{s}^2$$
$$v = 8.86 \text{ m/s}$$

Questions

Q-80

Which of the following is not an example of an oxidation-reduction reaction?

(A) combustion of wood

(B) rusting of iron

(C) cellular respiration

(D) electrolysis of water

Your Answer _____

Q-81

In the periodic table, what will an element on the left side of a row have a lower amount of than an element on the right side of the same row?

(A) density

(B) viscosity

(C) mass

(D) atomic number

Your Answer _____

Correct Answers

A–80

(D) Electrolysis of water is not an example of an oxidation-reduction reaction because it is an example of a decomposition reaction. Combustion of wood, rusting of iron, and cellular respiration are all examples of oxidation-reduction reactions.

A–81

(D) Elements on the left side of a row will have a lower atomic number than elements on the right side of the same row. The atomic number is the number of protons in an atom's nucleus. Density is a characteristic defined by mass per unit volume. Viscosity is a fluid's resistance to flow. Mass is a measure of the quantity of matter. The periodic table does not provide information on an element's density, viscosity, or mass.

Questions

Q–82

Which of these is not an example of a solution?

(A) air

(B) soda water

(C) elemental gold

(D) dental-filling alloy

Your Answer _____

_____

Q–83

The concentration of a saltwater solution that causes a human blood cell to swell in size is best described as

(A) hypertonic

(B) isotonic

(C) hypotonic

(D) saturated

Your Answer _____

_____

Correct Answers

A–82

(C) Elemental gold it not an example of a solution, since it is made of a single substance. A solution is a homogenous mixture of two or more substances, consisting of ions or molecules. Solutions can exist as solids, liquids, or gases. Air is a gaseous solution composed of nitrogen, oxygen, water vapor, and other gases. Soda water is a liquid solution composed of carbon dioxide dissolved in water. Dental-filling alloy is a solid solution often made of mercury, silver, and other metals.

A–83

(C) Salt is not permeable to the human blood cell membrane; therefore, the cell reaches equilibrium through osmosis. Swelling occurs because water is entering the cell through osmosis. This means that the concentration of salt inside the cell is greater than the concentration of salt outside the cell. The lower concentration of salt outside the cell is called a hypotonic solution ("hypo" = "low") and is the correct answer. The higher concentration of salt inside the cell is called a hypertonic solution ("hyper" = "high"). Isotonic means an equal concentration of salt both inside and outside the cell. A saturated solution refers to a solution with the maximum amount of salt dissolved in it and does not describe this situation.

Questions

Julie and Tom are studying for their nursing exam across from each other at a wide table in the library. Julie slides a 3.1 kg textbook toward Tom. If the net external force acting on the book is 4.1 N to the right, what is the book's acceleration?

(A)   0.8 m/s^2 to the right

(B)   1.3 m/s^2 to the right

(C)   7.2 m/s^2 to the right

(D)   12.7 m/s^2 to the right

Your Answer _____

_____

Correct Answers

A–84

(B)   Newton's second law states that the acceleration of an object is directly proportional to the net external force acting on the object and inversely proportional to the object's mass. In equation form, this law can be written as

$$\Sigma F = ma$$
net external force = mass $\times$ acceleration

Since the unknown is the acceleration, the equation can be written as

$$a = \Sigma F/m$$

The net external force on the book is 4.1 N to the right, and the mass of the book is 3.1 kg. Therefore, the acceleration is

$$a = 4.1 \text{ N}/3.1 \text{ kg}$$
$$a = 1.3 \text{ m/s}^2 \text{ to the right}$$

It is important to note that acceleration has both magnitude and direction.

Questions

Q–85

The temperature outside the hospital is 32°C. What is the temperature using the Fahrenheit scale?

(A) 57.6°F

(B) 17.8°F

(C) 49.8°F

(D) 89.6°F

Your Answer _____

Q–86

Which of the following represents the correct order of gene expression?

(A) RNA → DNA → Protein

(B) Protein → DNA → RNA

(C) DNA → Protein → RNA

(D) DNA → RNA → Protein

Your Answer _____

Correct Answers

A-85

(D)   Celsius and Fahrenheit temperature measurements can be converted to each other using the following equation:

$$T_F = \tfrac{9}{5} T_C + 32.0$$

Fahrenheit temperature

$$= (\tfrac{9}{5} \times \text{Celsius temperature}) + 32.0$$

The given temperature was 32°C. Converting this temperature to Fahrenheit

$$T_F = (\tfrac{9}{5} \times 32°\text{C}) + 32$$
$$T_F = (57.6°) + 32$$
$$T_F = 89.6°\text{F}$$

A-86

(D)   Gene expression begins in the nucleus through the process of transcription, where the information of DNA is used to construct an mRNA sequence. This mRNA sequence travels out of the nucleus and into the cytoplasm. Here, the ribosome completes the process of translation, where the information from the mRNA transcript is used to produce a sequence of amino acids or protein.

Questions

Q–87

As suggested by their position in the periodic table, what do the elements magnesium (Mg) and barium (Ba) have in common?

(A) They are in the same period.

(B) They have the same number of valence electrons.

(C) They are both liquids at room temperature.

(D) They have the same atomic mass.

Your Answer _____

_____

Q–88

Bill and Jodi walk to work at the hospital every morning. If they walk at an average speed of 0.95 m/s, and the hospital is 1.3 miles away, how long does it take them to get to the hospital?

(A) 36.5 minutes

(B) 82.1 minutes

(C) 32.9 minutes

(D) 74.1 minutes

Your Answer _____

_____

Correct Answers

A–87

(B) Magnesium and barium have the same number of valence electrons, a property that generally applies to elements in the same group, or column, on the periodic table. These two elements do not share the same period, or row. Magnesium and barium are both solids at room temperature. Barium's atomic mass is more than five times larger than magnesium's atomic mass.

A–88

(A) One mile is equal to approximately 1.6 km, or 1600 meters. Therefore, 1.3 miles is equal to approximately 2080 meters. Using the equation for average velocity:

$$V_{avg} = \Delta x/\Delta t$$
$$\text{Average Velocity} = \text{Displacement/Time}$$

results in:

$$0.95 \text{ m/s} = (2080 \text{ m})/\Delta t$$

therefore:

$$\Delta t = (2{,}080 \text{ m})/(0.95 \text{ m/s})$$
$$\Delta t = 2{,}189.47 \text{ s}$$

Since all of the potential answer choices are in minutes, the time needs to be converted to minutes by dividing by 60:

$$\Delta t = (2{,}189.47 \text{ s})/(60 \text{ s/min})$$
$$\Delta t = 36.5 \text{ minutes}$$

Questions

A step-up transformer is used on a 120 V line to provide a potential difference of 2,000 V. If the primary winding has 45 turns, how many turns does the secondary winding have?

(A)   27 turns

(B)   5,333 turns

(C)   45 turns

(D)   750 turns

Your Answer _____

_____

Correct Answers

(D) In its simplest form, an electric transformer consists of two coils of wire wound around a core of soft iron. One coil is connected to the input potential difference source. This is called the primary winding. The other coil, called the secondary winding, is connected to the output potential difference. Because the strength of the magnetic field and the cross-sectional area of the iron core is the same for both the primary and secondary winding, the potential differences across the two windings differ only because of the different number of turns of wire in each. This relationship is given by:

$$\Delta V_2 = (N_2/N_1)\Delta V_1$$

Potential Difference in Secondary
= (Number of Turns in Secondary/
Number of Turns in Primary)
× Potential Difference in Primary

For an input of 120 V onto a primary winding of 45 turns to produce an output of 2,000 V, the secondary winding must have:

$$2{,}000 \text{ V} = (N_2/45) \times 120 \text{ V}$$
$$N_2 = 750 \text{ turns}$$

Questions

Q–90

People perceive sound differently underwater than they do in air. Which of the following correctly describes the motion of sound waves in air and in water?

(A) Sound waves travel faster in air than in water.

(B) Sound waves travel slower in air than in water.

(C) Sound waves cannot travel in water.

(D) Sound waves travel at the same speed in air and in water.

Your Answer _____

_____

Q–91

A 20 kg box sits on the floor next to a wall. A person pushes on the box to the right toward the wall with a force of 150 N. Which of the following statements about this situation is true?

(A) The floor pushes 150 N up on the box.

(B) The box pushes 150 N down on the floor.

(C) The wall pushes 150 N to the left on the box.

(D) The wall does not push on the box.

Your Answer _____

_____

Correct Answers

A–90

(B) Sound waves can travel through solids, liquids, and gases. Because waves consist of particle vibrations, the speed of a sound wave depends on how quickly one particle can transfer its motion from one particle to another. The closer the particles are to each other, the faster the transfer of motion will be. Because the particles in water are closer together than they are in air, sound waves travel slower in air than in water. The speed of sound in air at 25°C is approximately 346 m/s, while the speed of sound in water at 25°C is approximately 1,490 m/s.

A–91

(C) Newton's third law states that if two objects interact, the magnitude of the force exerted on object 1 by object 2 is equal to the magnitude of the force simultaneously exerted on object 2 by object 1, and these two forces are opposite in direction. As the box is exerting a force of 150 N against the wall to the right, the wall is exerting a force of 150 N against the box to the left.

Questions

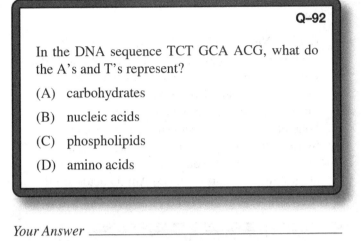

Q–92

In the DNA sequence TCT GCA ACG, what do the A's and T's represent?

(A) carbohydrates

(B) nucleic acids

(C) phospholipids

(D) amino acids

Your Answer _____

_____

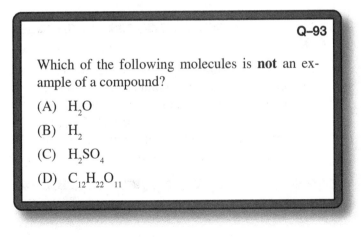

Q–93

Which of the following molecules is **not** an example of a compound?

(A) H_2O

(B) H_2

(C) H_2SO_4

(D) $C_{12}H_{22}O_{11}$

Your Answer _____

_____

Correct Answers

A–92

(B) Nucleic acids is the correct answer. There are four nucleic acids found in DNA: adenine, thiamine, guanine and cytosine. While (C) phospholipids and (A) carbohydrates are found in the DNA molecule, they compose the sugar phosphate backbone of the DNA molecule and are not represented by the letters A, T, C, and G. In addition, histone proteins are found around the DNA molecule, but are not directly part of it. (D) Amino acids are the building blocks of proteins such as histones.

A–93

(B) H_2, or hydrogen gas, is a molecule that is not a compound, because compounds are defined as substances with atoms of two or more different elements bound together. H_2O (water), H_2SO_4 (battery acid), and $C_{12}H_{22}O_{11}$ (table sugar) all fit this definition, so they are all compounds.

Questions

Q–94

Two animals of different species would be least likely to

(A) have similar anatomy

(B) compete for similar resources

(C) produce viable offspring

(D) occupy the same ecological niche

Your Answer _____

Q–95

Organic chemistry is defined as the study of compounds containing which element?

(A) oxygen

(B) hydrogen

(C) carbon

(D) nitrogen

Your Answer _____

Correct Answers

A–94

(C)   Different species have different numbers and different amounts of genes on their chromosomes. Two different species would not be likely to produce viable offspring because their chromosomes and genes would not correspond during meiosis. The other choices are plausible. (A) Different organisms may have similar anatomical structures (monkey's and human's arms), (B) may compete for similar resources (two species of shark with certain species of fish), and (D) may occupy the same ecological niche (like some species of birds that use other birds' nests).

A–95

(C)   Organic chemistry is defined as the study of compounds containing carbon. Compounds containing oxygen, hydrogen, and nitrogen, but not carbon, are not organic compounds and are not studied as part of organic chemistry.

Questions

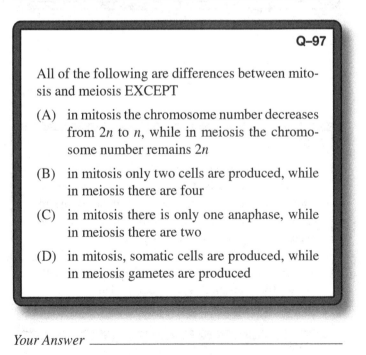

Q-96

A cat sitting on a pier looks into the water and sees a fish. To the cat, the fish appears to be larger and closer to the water's surface than it actually is. This change in appearance is due to

(A) refraction of the light waves

(B) interference of the water and the light waves

(C) diffraction of the light waves

(D) polarization of the light waves

Your Answer _____

Q-97

All of the following are differences between mitosis and meiosis EXCEPT

(A) in mitosis the chromosome number decreases from $2n$ to n, while in meiosis the chromosome number remains $2n$

(B) in mitosis only two cells are produced, while in meiosis there are four

(C) in mitosis there is only one anaphase, while in meiosis there are two

(D) in mitosis, somatic cells are produced, while in meiosis gametes are produced

Your Answer _____

Correct Answers

A–96

(A) The speed of light is slower as it travels in a substance than it is when it travels in a vacuum. This ratio of the speed of light in a vacuum to the speed of light in a medium is known as the medium's index of refraction. The higher the index of refraction, the slower the speed of light is as it travels through the medium. As the light passes from the air, which has a low index of refraction, into the water, which has a higher index of refraction, the light rays are bent toward the normal. This bending of the light rays causes the image of the fish to appear to be closer to the surface than it actually is. Because it appears closer, it also appears larger.

A–97

(A) All of the statements are correct EXCEPT (A). During mitosis, the chromosome number remains $2n$. Since the purpose of mitosis is the reproduction of somatic cells, all chromosomes are necessary. During meiosis (oogenesis or spermatogenesis), the chromosome number is reduced to n in preparation for fertilization. When two gametes meet—for example, a sperm cell and an egg cell—the chromosome number returns to $2n$.

Questions

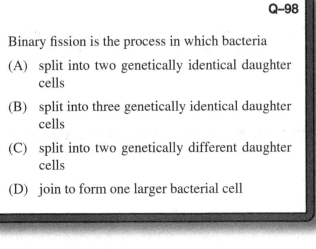

Q-98

Binary fission is the process in which bacteria

(A) split into two genetically identical daughter cells

(B) split into three genetically identical daughter cells

(C) split into two genetically different daughter cells

(D) join to form one larger bacterial cell

Your Answer _____

_____

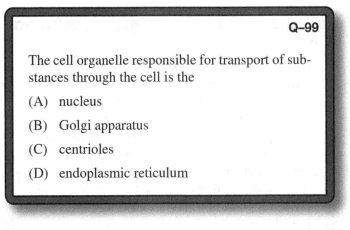

Q-99

The cell organelle responsible for transport of substances through the cell is the

(A) nucleus

(B) Golgi apparatus

(C) centrioles

(D) endoplasmic reticulum

Your Answer _____

_____

Correct Answers

A–98

(A) When binary fission occurs, two cells are produced, each with an identical set of bacterial chromosomes. The other answers are incorrect.

A–99

(D) Endoplasmic reticulum is the correct answer. The endoplasmic reticulum connects the nucleus and cytoplasm, facilitating gene expression as mRNA is transported from the nucleus to the ribosome. (A) The nucleus is the control center of the cell and directs cellular activities. (B) The Golgi apparatus stores and packages chemicals in the cell. (C) Centrioles secrete spindle fibers that assist with the separation of chromosomes in cellular division.

Questions

Q–100

Sea otters eat sea urchins. Sea urchins eat kelp, a type of brown algae. What might be the short-term effect on the ecosystem if great numbers of sea otters were removed from this environment?

(A) increase in sea urchin population, decrease in kelp population

(B) decrease in sea urchin population, increase in kelp population

(C) increase in sea urchin population, increase in kelp population

(D) decrease in sea urchin population, decrease in kelp population

Your Answer _____

_____

Q–101

By what types of bonds are compounds composed of two nonmetals likely to be held together?

(A) covalent

(B) compound

(C) ionic

(D) hydrogen

Your Answer _____

_____

Correct Answers

A–100

(A) With fewer sea otters, fewer sea urchins will be eaten. Therefore, the sea urchin population will increase. With more sea urchins, more kelp will be eaten, causing a decrease in the kelp population. (B), (C), and (D) are incorrect.

A–101

(A) Two nonmetals are usually held together by covalent bonds, in which atoms share electrons. A compound is a substance made of atoms of two or more different elements bound together, not a type of bond. An ionic bond usually forms between metals and nonmetals. Hydrogen bonds, which are weak bonds in which a hydrogen atom bound to a highly electronegative element in a given molecule and a second highly electronegative atom in another molecule or elsewhere in the same molecule, are not the most likely way through which two nonmetals are held together.

Questions

Q-102

Benzene, a hydrocarbon that is a natural part of crude oil, has the chemical formula C_6H_6. What shape is this molecule?

(A) square

(B) ring

(C) linear

(D) triangle

Your Answer _____

_____

Q-103

All of the following will eventually denature enzymes EXCEPT

(A) increased temperature

(B) decreased temperature

(C) increased pH

(D) decreased pH

Your Answer _____

_____

Correct Answers

A–102

(B) Benzene molecules have a ring shape. Other hydrocarbons, such as cyclobutane, have a square-shaped structure. Alkanes are simple, linear hydrocarbons. Cyclopropane is a triangle-shaped hydrocarbon.

A–103

(B) Although increasing the temperature of an enzyme will initially increase the activity of the enzyme, eventually it will denature. Similarly, increasing the pH (making a solution more basic) and decreasing the pH (making a solution more acidic) will denature the enzyme. Decreasing the temperature of the enzyme reduces the molecular kinetics of the enzyme, but does not denature it. As the temperature falls, the random movement of the enzyme and its frequency of contact with the substrate decreases, causing the rate of the enzymatic reaction to slow.

Questions

Q–104

The phenotypes of a heterozygous white-haired female rabbit and a homozygous white-haired male rabbit are

(A) Ww and WW

(B) white

(C) gray

(D) black

Your Answer _____

Q–105

A bowling ball, with a mass of 8 kg, has a kinetic energy level of 36 joules. At what speed is the bowling ball moving?

(A) 9.0 m/s

(B) 4.5 m/s

(C) 3.0 m/s

(D) 1.5 m/s

Your Answer _____

Correct Answers

A–104

(B)   The phenotype of both rabbits described is white. (A) is incorrect because it represents the genotypes of the two rabbits. (C) and (D) are incorrect because they represent phenotypes of rabbits other than those presented in the question.

A–105

(C)   Kinetic energy is related to the mass and the velocity of the object. This relationship is given by the expression $KE = \frac{1}{2}mv^2$. Using the given information, 36 joules $= \frac{1}{2}(8 \text{ kg})v^2$. This would result in $v^2 = 9 \text{ m}^2/\text{s}^2$, and $v = 3$ m/s. It is important to note that in the kinetic energy equation, the velocity is squared. Therefore, in order to find the velocity, the square root of the result must be calculated.

Questions

Unlike solids or liquids, gases can change in volume. How does Boyle's law state that the volume of a gas at a given temperature varies with the applied pressure?

(A) inversely

(B) conversely

(C) continuously

(D) equally

Your Answer _____

_____

Correct Answers

A–106

(A) Boyle's law states that the volume of gas at a given temperature varies inversely with the applied pressure. Volume cannot vary conversely, continuously, or equally with the applied pressure.

Questions

Q–107

Which of the following correctly traces a drop of blood from the superior vena cava through the heart to the aorta?

(A) superior vena cava → left atrium → left ventricle → pulmonary artery → lungs → pulmonary vein → right atrium → right ventricle → aorta

(B) superior vena cava → left atrium → left ventricle → pulmonary vein → lungs → pulmonary artery → right atrium → right ventricle → aorta

(C) superior vena cava → right atrium → right ventricle → pulmonary artery → lungs → pulmonary vein → left atrium → left ventricle → aorta

(D) superior vena cava → right atrium → right ventricle → pulmonary vein → lungs → pulmonary artery → left atrium → left ventricle → aorta

Your Answer _____

_____

Correct Answers

A–107

(C) Deoxygenated blood enters from the superior vena cava to the left atrium and passes through the tricuspid valve to the left ventricle. Blood is then pumped through the pulmonary valve to the pulmonary vein before entering the lungs and becoming re-oxygenated. Blood returns through the left atrium, passes through the mitral valve, and enters the left ventricle. Finally, the oxygenated blood is pumped out of the aortic valve and out of the heart. (A), (B), and (D) are incorrect.

Questions

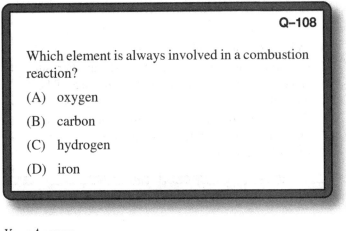

Q-108

Which element is always involved in a combustion reaction?

(A) oxygen

(B) carbon

(C) hydrogen

(D) iron

Your Answer _____

_____

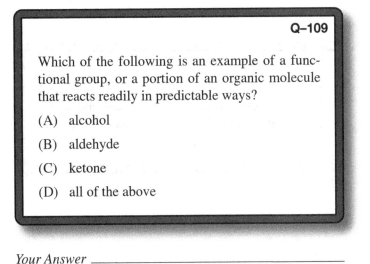

Q-109

Which of the following is an example of a functional group, or a portion of an organic molecule that reacts readily in predictable ways?

(A) alcohol

(B) aldehyde

(C) ketone

(D) all of the above

Your Answer _____

_____

Correct Answers

A–108

(A) Oxygen is always involved in combustion reaction. This element reacts with another substance, usually producing a rapid release of heat and a flame. Other elements, including carbon, hydrogen, and iron, can react with oxygen in a combustion reaction, but they are not necessary for this type of reaction to occur.

A–109

(D) Alcohols, aldehydes, and ketones are all functional groups. Most alcohols and aldehydes are readily oxidized. Aldehydes and ketones can be reduced to alcohols.

Questions

Q–110

The theory which states that new species develop through evolution rapidly at times such as ice ages or meteorite impacts, but remain stable otherwise, is known as

(A) gradualism

(B) adaptation

(C) punctuated equilibrium

(D) natural selection

Your Answer _____

_____

Correct Answers

A–110

(C) Punctuated equilibrium is one explanation for evolution; the theory holds that species undergo minor evolutionary changes until major events occur. During these major events, evolutionary change could lead to the development of many different species out of new geographic barriers, population bottlenecks, or other phenomenon. (A) Gradualism is a rival theory that suggests organisms are constantly evolving from generation to generation and speciation is a gradual process. (B) An adaptation is a trait that improves an organism's chance of survival and eventual reproduction. (D) Natural selection is the basic explanation for evolution where the most fit organisms are more likely to survive and reproduce more, influencing the next generation by passing on more of their traits to the population.

Questions

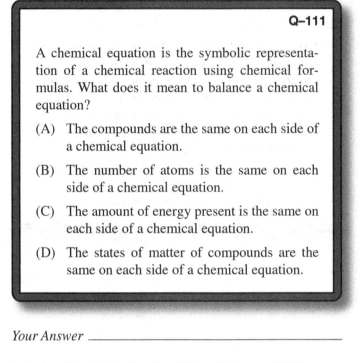

Q–111

A chemical equation is the symbolic representation of a chemical reaction using chemical formulas. What does it mean to balance a chemical equation?

(A) The compounds are the same on each side of a chemical equation.

(B) The number of atoms is the same on each side of a chemical equation.

(C) The amount of energy present is the same on each side of a chemical equation.

(D) The states of matter of compounds are the same on each side of a chemical equation.

Your Answer _____

_____

Correct Answers

A–111

(B) To balance a chemical equation is to make sure that the number of atoms is the same on each side of a chemical equation. Compounds will change through the course of a chemical reaction, so they will not be the same on each side of a chemical equation. Though energy is conserved in reactions in closed systems, this is not reflected in a chemical reaction. States of matter may change in the course of a chemical reaction, so they may not be the same on each side of a chemical equation.

Questions

Q–112

After leaving the stomach, which anatomical structure does food travel to first?

(A) duodenum

(B) ileum

(C) jejunum

(D) cecum

Your Answer _____

_____

Q–113

The arrows in a food web represent the

(A) direction organisms move in an environment

(B) direction of energy flow through a series of organisms

(C) order of importance of the various organisms

(D) return of chemicals to the environment

Your Answer _____

_____

Correct Answers

A–112

(A) Duodenum is the correct answer. The duodenum is the name of the first segment of the small intestine. It is connected to the stomach. (B) The ileum is the final section of the small intestine. (C) The jejunum is the middle section of the small intestine. (D) The cecum is the first segment of the large intestine.

A–113

(B) The arrows in a food web represent energy flow through a series of organisms. The arrows do not represent the direction of organism movement in an ecosystem (A). A food web has nothing to do with the importance of an organism, as indicated by (C), or how chemicals return to the environment, as indicated by (D). The purpose of a food web is to show relationships between organisms and to represent energy flow through an ecosystem.

Questions

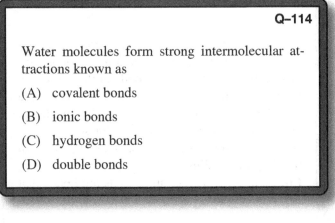

Q–114

Water molecules form strong intermolecular attractions known as

(A) covalent bonds

(B) ionic bonds

(C) hydrogen bonds

(D) double bonds

Your Answer _____

_____

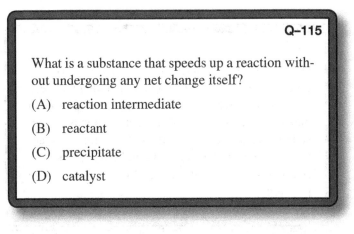

Q–115

What is a substance that speeds up a reaction without undergoing any net change itself?

(A) reaction intermediate

(B) reactant

(C) precipitate

(D) catalyst

Your Answer _____

_____

Correct Answers

A–114

(C)   Water molecules form strong intermolecular attractions known as hydrogen bonds. Hydrogen bonds are not true bonds in the sense that they do not link atoms or ions together. The word "bond" signifies the strength of the attractive force. Hydrogen bonds are responsible for some of water's unique properties, such as its relatively high melting and boiling points, and surface tension. Covalent, ionic, and double bonds are bonds that link atoms or ions together.

A–115

(D)   A catalyst is a substance that speeds up a reaction without undergoing any net change itself. A reaction intermediate is a substance produced during a reaction that itself reacts in a subsequent step, so doesn't appear in the net equation. A reactant is a starting substance in a chemical reaction. A precipitate is a solid formed by a reaction in a solution.

Questions

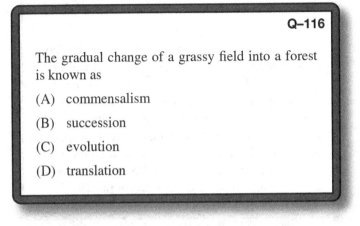

Q–116

The gradual change of a grassy field into a forest is known as

(A) commensalism

(B) succession

(C) evolution

(D) translation

Your Answer _____

_____

Q–117

In the Haber-Bosch process, a method for producing much of the nitrogen used for fertilizer, nitrogen gas, N_2, reacts with hydrogen gas to produce ammonia, or NH_3. The nitrogen atoms go from equally sharing electrons in nitrogen gas to acquiring a greater portion of shared electrons in ammonia. What word describes the process that occurs in each nitrogen atom?

(A) oxidation

(B) reduction

(C) ionization

(D) Haberization

Your Answer  _____

_____

Correct Answers

A–116

(B) Succession is the correct answer. The process of gradual change in an ecosystem from one type to another is referred to as succession. (A) Commensalism is a type of symbiosis in which one organism benefits and the other is neither helped nor harmed. (C) Evolution is the change of species over time. (D) Translation refers to the process of the information of messenger RNA being used to construct an amino acid sequence or protein.

A–117

(B) The process that occurs in each nitrogen atom as it goes from equally sharing electrons to acquiring a greater portion of shared electrons is reduction. Oxidation is the opposite process, where atoms lose a shared portion of electrons. Ionization is the condition of being dissociated into ions, which does not occur here. Haberization does not describe what happens to nitrogen atoms in the Haber-Bosch process.

Questions

Q–118

An ion is an atom or group of atoms with a charge. What is a cation?

(A) a positively charged atom or group of atoms

(B) a negatively charged atom or group of atoms

(C) an atom or group of atoms with no charge

(D) an atom or group of atoms derived from an ion

Your Answer _____

_____

Q–119

The design of an airplane's wings provides the lift needed to fly the airplane. This lift can be explained using which of the following principles?

(A) Pascal's principle

(B) Newton's principle

(C) Bernoulli's principle

(D) Archimedes' principle

Your Answer _____

_____

Correct Answers

A–118

(A) A cation is a positively charged atom. Metal atoms often form cations. A negatively charged atom is called an anion. Atoms with no charge are simply called atoms. A cation is not derived from an ion.

A–119

(C) The air flowing over an airplane's wings exhibits the same properties as a fluid in motion. Bernoulli's principle states that the pressure in a fluid decreases as the fluid's velocity increases. Airplane wings are designed such that the air speed above the wing is greater than the air speed below the wing. The increased air velocity on the top of the wing provides lower pressure on the top of the wing; thus, the higher pressure below the wing causes a net upward force on the wing. This causes the airplane to lift off the ground. Archimedes' principle and Pascal's principle are both related to fluid dynamics (Archimedes' principle dealing with buoyancy and Pascal's principle dealing with distribution of applied pressure in a closed container), but only Bernoulli's principle explains the lift of an airplane. While Newton was instrumental in the study and development of the field of physics, and was credited with developing Newton's laws of motion, he did not have a principle named after him.

Questions

Q-120

Since water is a polar molecule, compounds with which type of bonds are *more likely* to dissolve in water than compounds with other types of bonds?

(A) ionic

(B) hydrogen

(C) covalent

(D) carbon-carbon

Your Answer _____

Correct Answers

A–120

(A) Compounds with ionic bonds are more likely to dissolve in water than compounds with other types of bonds because the positive and negative ions are attracted to the oppositely charged ends of the water molecule. Hydrogen bonds do not link atoms or ions together, and do not affect a compound's dissolvability in water. Covalent bonds do not occur between charged particles, so compounds with covalent bonds are less likely to dissolve in water. Carbon-carbon bonds occur in many compounds and do not affect dissolvability in water.

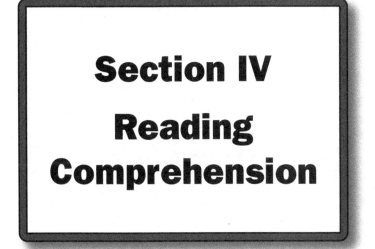

Section IV

Reading Comprehension

Passage 1

Read the following passage and answer Questions 1 to 8.

Why You Should Choose Biodiesel
Since the early part of the twentieth century, diesel has fueled the engines for many vehicles. In 1892, an inventor named Rudolf Diesel invented an engine that could use liquid coal dust as fuel. Diesel engines are a type of internal combustion engine in which heat created by air compression ignites liquid fuel. When fuel is injected into the combustion chambers, the air inside the diesel engine is hot enough to ignite the fuel instantly. In this way, unlike regular gasoline engines, which require spark plugs to ignite the air-fuel mixture, diesel engines do not require an intermediary device to begin the fuel ignition process. Diesel fuel is also less flammable and explosive than regular gasoline. These advantages make diesel the fuel of choice for military vehicles as well as commercial trucks and public transport vehicles. A major disadvantage of the traditional diesel engine is the production of sooty, smelly, black smoke.

Looking to nature for diesel alternatives
With the rough economy, volatile gas prices, and a potentially limited supply of fossil fuels, alternative energy sources are becoming increasingly popular as cheaper and more energy-efficient ways to meet our fuel needs. Biodiesel can be a viable alternative to petroleum diesel fuel. Made from natural sources, biodiesel is biodegradable, made from renewable oils, free of sulfur and aromatics, and thus is cleaner for the environment.

Over the past 15 years, biodiesel has become more popular globally due to its many perceived benefits. Through a basic refining process, biodiesel can be made from any number of renewable fats and oils, including vegetable, canola, and peanut oils. Because soybeans are a major commodity grown and traded throughout the world, including 30 states in the United States, biodiesel can have a potentially global impact. Also, one of the by-products of the biodiesel refining process is glycerin, which can be used in a host of products, including toothpaste and plastic.

Other advantages to biodiesel include less wear and tear on existing engines and fuel equipment, as well as greater fuel and operating efficiency. Biodiesel can be used seamlessly in petroleum diesel vehicles with few

(Continued)

engine modifications. Indeed, when blended at a 20% rate with petroleum diesel, biodiesel has improved lubricity and less engine wear than regular gasoline, improving the overall life span of an engine through its superior lubricating properties. Additionally, unlike other alternative fuels, it is possible to store and dispense biodiesel anywhere, since it can easily be blended with petroleum diesel.

Research suggests that biodiesel is a useful alternative fuel for niche markets, such as urban transport vehicles and the commercial or recreational marine industry, which make up around 10% of the overall petroleum diesel in the United States.

Minimizing environmental impact

Although it is easy to store, biodiesel degrades about four times faster than petroleum fuel, only without any of the latter's characteristic smelly, toxic emissions. In a sense, biodiesel is the ideal fuel because it is biodegradable, non-toxic, and virtually free of sulfur and aromatics. Using biodiesel and biodiesel fuel blends can be advantageous for large urban areas or confined spaces because of its less offensive exhaust odor, reduced pollutants, and minimal eye irritants.

Biodiesel also directly helps Earth through releasing fewer pollutants, such as carbon dioxide, hydrocarbons, and sulfurous compounds. One major advantage of biodiesel is that it reduces the major greenhouse gas components in the atmosphere, including carbon dioxide, carbon monoxide, and hazardous diesel particulate. This means that biodiesel actually helps to prevent depletion of the ozone layer and acid rain rather than contribute to it.

On the other hand, conventional petroleum diesel has an extremely negative environmental impact because it releases hydrocarbons, which are a major source of pollution in sensitive places like large urban areas, lakes, and inland waterways. Indeed, many freshwater lakes in the United States have been so affected by acid rain and other environmental pollutants that entire marine populations have been destroyed. Another problem for cities is that the output of sulfurous compounds, especially sulfuric acid, from petroleum diesel can damage limestone and marble on valuable buildings and historic sites.

The costs of biodiesel

Despite its advantages, biodiesel fuel is not without its costs and performance effects. The price of biodiesel is dependent on the market price for oils. Biodiesel-petroleum blends can cost 15 to 30 cents per gallon more than petroleum diesel alone.

The high cost of biodiesel makes it ideal for niche markets for which a cleaner, biodegradable fuel is important. Indeed, research suggests that biodiesel is a useful alternative fuel for niche markets, such as urban transport vehicles and the commercial or recreational marine industry, which make up around 10% of the overall petroleum diesel in the United States. However, costs for biodiesel could decrease if more arable land was devoted to growing ingredients for biodiesel.

Other roadblocks for biodiesel's use in conventional vehicles include concerns about engine performance and overall sustainability. Due to its high concentration of unsaturated fatty compounds, vegetable oil reacts with oxygen then petroleum diesel, which means that it can leave more unwanted, gummy deposits in engines than regular diesel. Similarly, biodiesel has a higher gel point than regular diesel, which means that it is more susceptible to freezing. Although some of these obstacles can be overcome with more efficient engine technology, such as special heaters or through increased use of biodiesel-petroleum diesel blends, more research needs to be done before you'll see many of your neighbors driving biodiesel cars to the grocery store.

Nevertheless, due to its cleaner emissions, favorable odor, and minimal environmental impact, biodiesel seems an obvious choice over petroleum diesel as a way to maintain our fuel supply in a way that will minimize climate change.

Questions

Q–1

In the first paragraph, the author suggests that spark plugs

(A) contribute to environmental pollution through the release of harmful fumes

(B) interfere with the composition of the air-fuel mixture in gasoline engines

(C) make gasoline engines less efficient than diesel engines

(D) produce air that is too cool to be used in diesel engines

Your Answer _____

_____

Q–2

In the **Looking to nature for diesel alternatives** section, the author's use of the phrase "viable alternative" suggests that petroleum diesel fuel

(A) comes from chemical, rather than natural, sources

(B) contains toxins and other harmful substances

(C) is designed to be a long-lasting substance

(D) is used infrequently across the world

Your Answer _____

_____

Correct Answers

A–1

(C) The author's description of how gasoline engines work suggests that spark plugs are an extra step in the fuel combustion process that does not exist in diesel engines. This implies that spark plugs make gasoline engines more inefficient, which makes (C) the correct answer. Gasoline engines and regular diesel engines both release harmful fumes into the environment, so (A) is incorrect. Similarly, there is no suggestion that spark plugs either interfere with the composition of the air-fuel mixture in gasoline engines, as (B) states, or produce air that is too cool for diesel engines, as in (D).

A–2

(B) The author's description of biodiesel as a "viable alternative" to petroleum diesel suggests that petroleum diesel fuel contains impurities and other substances that are toxic to the environment. Nevertheless, (A) is incorrect. This section does not suggest that petroleum derives from chemical sources, but rather that it is less naturally pure than biodiesel. Also, (C) and (D) are incorrect, since there is no suggestion that petroleum diesel is purposefully designed to be longer lasting or that it somehow is used less frequently because of the increase in use of biodiesel.

Questions

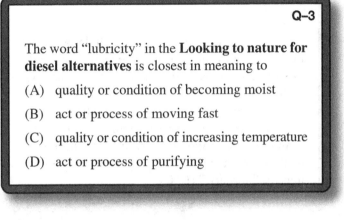

Q–3

The word "lubricity" in the **Looking to nature for diesel alternatives** is closest in meaning to

(A) quality or condition of becoming moist

(B) act or process of moving fast

(C) quality or condition of increasing temperature

(D) act or process of purifying

Your Answer _____

_____

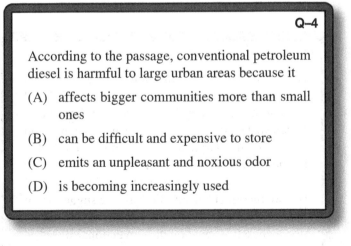

Q–4

According to the passage, conventional petroleum diesel is harmful to large urban areas because it

(A) affects bigger communities more than small ones

(B) can be difficult and expensive to store

(C) emits an unpleasant and noxious odor

(D) is becoming increasingly used

Your Answer _____

_____

Correct Answers

A–3

(A) The word "lubricity," which derives from the word "lubricate," means "the quality or condition of being moist." So (A) is the correct answer. Although the author describes the process of refining biodiesel, which makes (D) an attractive answer, this is not a correct meaning of "lubricity." Similarly, while moving fast and heating up are qualities of an engine, these are not correct meanings of "lubricity." (B, C)

A–4

(C) In the passage, the author suggests that the foul-smelling emissions from conventional diesel are particularly dangerous to large urban areas, which makes (C) the correct answer. There is no suggestion that large urban areas are more affected by the pollution from conventional diesel than are smaller communities, as in (A). Similarly, (B) and (D) are incorrect because the passage suggests that biodiesel is, in fact, more expensive than conventional diesel, even though conventional diesel is used less nowadays.

Questions

Q–5

The word "niche" in **The costs of biodiesel** section is closest in meaning to

(A) select

(B) gracious

(C) important

(D) expensive

Your Answer _____

_____

Q–6

According to the passage, what is one reason biodiesel is slow to be incorporated into everyday vehicle engines?

(A) Its environmental effects remain uncertain.

(B) It is too expensive for researchers to test extensively.

(C) It is less adaptable to different types of vehicles than conventional diesel.

(D) Its constituent compounds are unstable and can cause engine deposits.

Your Answer _____

_____

Correct Answers

A–5

(A) The word "niche" means "select" or "target," so (A) is the correct answer. Although "niche" resembles the word "nice," which makes (B) an attractive answer, this is not the correct meaning of the given word. Similarly, while the author describes the benefits and costs of biodiesel, which makes (C) and (D) attractive answers, these are not correct meanings of the word "niche."

A–6

(D) This question requires a correct inference from the final paragraphs of the passage, so (D) is the correct answer. In this section, the author implies that more research needs to be done to improve the usability of biodiesel in normal vehicles because of the unstable, fatty nature of the oils and also its tendency to leave deposits. Although biodiesel is a relatively newer concept than conventional diesel, which makes (A), (B), and (C) attractive answers, its positive environmental effects are well documented, as are its accessibility for research and its adaptability in different types of vehicles.

Questions

Q-7

Which of the following would be another appropriate title for this passage?

(A) Creative Ways to Improve Your Engine's Performance

(B) Alternative Fuels: Friend or Foe?

(C) Alternative Fuels for Your Health and Your World

(D) Are Environmental Pollutants Really Dangerous?

Your Answer _____

_____

Q-8

The author's primary purpose in writing this passage is to

(A) inform readers with research data about the effects of biodiesel

(B) describe for readers different stages in the development of biodiesel

(C) entertain readers by relating stories about the development of biodiesel

(D) persuade readers with informed arguments about the effects of biodiesel

Your Answer _____

_____

Correct Answers

A–7

(C)   The best alternative title for this passage should correctly summarize the main idea of the passage. So, the correct answer is (C) because it is an accurate summary. In this article, the author analyzes the benefits and costs of biodiesel to support the positive impact of alternative fuels. (A), (B), and (D) address minor themes in the passage but do not fully encompass the main idea.

A–8

(D)   The title of this passage, "Why You Should Choose Biodiesel," marks this article as a persuasive piece, so (D) is the correct answer. Although the reader is informed and entertained with information throughout the article, an approach that makes (A), (B), and (C) attractive answers, these are not the author's primary purpose or main plan in writing this article.

Passage 2

Read the following passage and answer Questions 9 to 19.

Chicken and Rice Soup

Ready to Serve. Do Not Add Water.

Stovetop: Heat in 1-quart saucepan until hot, stirring occasionally.

Microwave: Heat in covered microwavable bowl on **High 3–5 minutes** until hot, stirring once. **Careful**—leave in microwave 1 minute; stir.

Ingredients: Chicken Broth (water, chicken stock, sea salt)*, **Carrots*, Cooked Chicken Meat*, Brown Rice*, Celery*. Contains Less than 1% of:** Corn Starch*, Sea Salt, Water, Chicken Flavor, Carrot Puree*, Chicken Fat*, Onion Powder, Soy Protein Concentrate, Black Pepper, Garlic, Chives, Rosemary, Yeast Extract, Potato Flour, Canola Oil.   *Organic

CONTAINS SOY INGREDIENTS

Nutrition Facts Serving Size 1 cup (245 g) Servings Per Container about 2	
Amount Per Serving	
Calories 100	Calories from Fat 15
	% Daily Value*
Total Fat 1.5 g	2%
Saturated Fat 0.5 g	3%
Trans Fat 0 g	
Polyunsaturated Fat 0.5 g	
Monounsaturated Fat 0.5 g	
Cholesterol 10 mg	3%
Sodium 600 mg	25%
Total Carbohydrate 12 g	4%
Dietary Fiber 1 g	4%
Sugars 1 g	
Protein 5 g	
Vitamin A 10%	Vitamin C 0%
Calcium 0%	Iron 0%
*Percent Daily Values are based on a 2,000 calorie diet	

Questions

Q–9

What does the author's use of the phrase "Do Not Add Water" suggest?

(A) The soup is made from natural ingredients that do not combine well with water.

(B) The soup is not condensed like other types of soup, so water is not necessary.

(C) The soup requires milk to complete the recipe, rather than water.

(D) The soup does not need water until after it has been heated.

Your Answer _____

_____

Correct Answers

A–9

(B) The soup label states that the soup is "ready to serve," which suggests that no additional ingredients are necessary. Although the soup is made from natural ingredients, as (A) suggests, this is not the reason that one should not add water. Similarly, while some cream-based soups require the addition of milk, this is not the case for this soup. So, (C) is incorrect. Also, while the soup does need to be heated, (D) is incorrect because water is completely unnecessary for preparing this soup.

Questions

Q-10

Why are separate directions *most likely* included in the soup recipe for stovetop and microwave preparation?

(A) Heating soup on a stovetop is more danger-ous than heating soup in a microwave.

(B) The soup company is legally required to de-scribe the different possible ways of heating the soup.

(C) Each cooking method requires different heat-ing techniques in order to achieve similar end results.

(D) Kitchen appliances, such as stovetops and microwaves, are often unreliable in heating substances.

Your Answer _____

_____

Correct Answers

A–10

(C)   Soup manufacturers include directions to show consumers how to achieve optimal results for heating the soup via common kitchen appliances. While kitchen appliances can be dangerous, as (A) suggests, this is not the reason the label includes separate stovetop and microwave instructions. Similarly, while soup manufacturers are required to include certain information on labels, as (B) states, this is not the main reason the separate directions were included. Finally, though kitchen appliances can be unreliable, as (D) suggests, this is not the main reason both stovetop and microwave directions are included on the label.

Questions

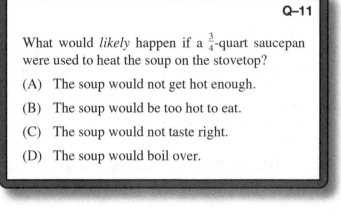

Q–11

What would *likely* happen if a $\frac{3}{4}$-quart saucepan were used to heat the soup on the stovetop?

(A) The soup would not get hot enough.

(B) The soup would be too hot to eat.

(C) The soup would not taste right.

(D) The soup would boil over.

Your Answer _____

_____

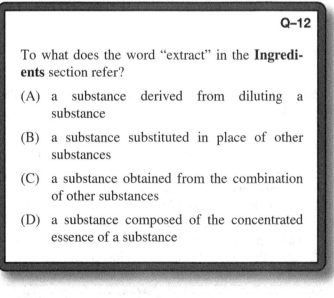

Q–12

To what does the word "extract" in the **Ingredients** section refer?

(A) a substance derived from diluting a substance

(B) a substance substituted in place of other substances

(C) a substance obtained from the combination of other substances

(D) a substance composed of the concentrated essence of a substance

Your Answer _____

_____

425

Correct Answers

A–11

(D) If a smaller saucepan were used to heat the soup, it would likely boil over because there would not be enough room in the saucepan for it to cook properly. In this way, (A), (B), and (C) are incorrect because there is no indication that using a smaller saucepan would adversely affect the soup's capacity to be heated, its edibleness, or its taste.

A–12

(D) An "extract" is a solution, often a liquid, made up of the concentrated essence of a particular substance, such as vanilla. Option (A) is incorrect because this describes how condensed substances are cooked. Option (B) refers to a "substitute" rather than an "extract," so it is incorrect. Similarly, option (C) refers to a "mixture" or "mélange" rather than an "extract," so it is incorrect.

Questions

Q–13

Why are specific words *most likely* bolded on the label?

(A) to illustrate for the consumer why this soup is a better product than other brands of soup

(B) to highlight interesting health and wellness information that the consumer may want to read

(C) to point out critical nutritional and preparation information that may affect the consumer's health

(D) to show the consumer that the manufacturer is attentive to presenting the soup in an attractive way

Your Answer _____

_____

Correct Answers

A–13

(C)   Words on the label are included in bold to highlight important nutritional and preparation information. While manufacturers are concerned with differentiating their brand from other types of soup and making their own soup appear attractive when creating labels, as (A) and (D) suggest, this is not the reason words are included in bold. Similarly, while the label does contain information that some consumers may find interesting, as (C) states, this is not the main reason the words are bolded on the label.

Questions

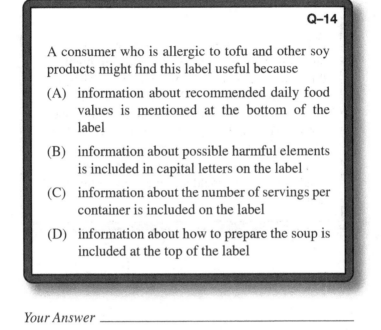

Q–14

A consumer who is allergic to tofu and other soy products might find this label useful because

(A) information about recommended daily food values is mentioned at the bottom of the label

(B) information about possible harmful elements is included in capital letters on the label

(C) information about the number of servings per container is included on the label

(D) information about how to prepare the soup is included at the top of the label

Your Answer _____

_____

Correct Answers

A–14

(B) The label includes a statement that it contains soy ingredients in capital letters to highlight this information for people with food allergies. While people with food allergies may generally be concerned with recommended daily food values, serving size, and preparation techniques, options (A), (C), and (D) are incorrect because they do not describe the most relevant reasons a person who is allergic to soy would specifically find this label helpful.

Questions

What information in the **Nutrition Facts** section would a person watching his or her salt intake find important?

(A) One serving of soup consists of one cup or 245 g of this product.

(B) One serving of soup has one-tenth of the recommended daily value of calcium.

(C) One serving of soup contains 100 calories, 15 of which are calories derived from fat.

(D) One serving of soup constitutes one-fourth of the recommended daily value of sodium.

Your Answer _____

_____

Correct Answers

A–15

(D) A person concerned about salt intake would need to pay attention to the fact that one serving of soup contains 25%, or one-fourth, of a person's recommended daily value of sodium. While a person watching his or her salt intake might be generally concerned about portion size, mineral intake, and fat, options (A), (B), and (C) are incorrect because they do not relate specifically to the amount of salt in the soup.

Questions

Read the following paragraph.

Polyunsaturated fats are fatty acids that have at least two double bonds in the representative molecule. On the other hand, monounsaturated fats are fatty acids that have a single double bond in the representative molecule.

Based on this paragraph and the passage, the prefix *poly-* most nearly means

(A) one

(B) none

(C) many

(D) select

Your Answer _____

_____

Correct Answers

A–16

(C)   The paragraph states that polyunsaturated fats have multiple double bonds, whereas monounsaturated fats have only one double bond, which suggests that "poly-" refers to "multiple" or "many." Option (A) is incorrect because the paragraph suggests that the prefix "mono-" means "one." Similarly, (B) and (D) are incorrect because the paragraph clearly states that polyunsaturated fats have at least two double bonds.

Questions

The use of asterisks to highlight organic ingredients on the label *mainly* suggests that the manufacturer

(A)   believes that consumers are concerned about knowing the origins of what they are buying

(B)   thinks that labeling its products as natural will stop consumers from buying other brands

(C)   finds that using natural substances makes its products cheaper for consumers to purchase

(D)   understands that consumers are attracted to buying products that seem expensive and exclusive

Your Answer _____

_____

Correct Answers

A–17

(A)   The manufacturer likely lists the organic ingredients to let consumers know that its products include many natural, chemical-free ingredients that are better for the consumers' health. Although the creation of food labels includes a degree of marketing awareness of competition, price structuring, and brand strategy, options (B), (C), and (D) are incorrect because they do not describe the *main* reason the manufacturer likely labels ingredients on the label as organic.

Questions

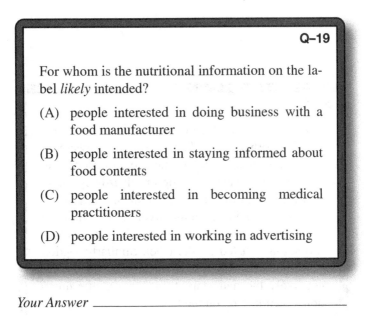

Q–18

What would be the most appropriate subheading to advertise this chicken rice soup?

(A) Ready to serve but do not add water

(B) Made with fresh vegetables and hormone-free chicken

(C) Heat quickly using stovetop and conventional microwave

(D) Contains chicken broth, cooked chicken, carrots, and sea salt

Your Answer _____

_____

Q–19

For whom is the nutritional information on the label *likely* intended?

(A) people interested in doing business with a food manufacturer

(B) people interested in staying informed about food contents

(C) people interested in becoming medical practitioners

(D) people interested in working in advertising

Your Answer _____

_____

Correct Answers

A–18

(B) An advertising slogan should include persuasive language. Since this product is mostly organic, the best subheading could be (B), as it promotes the soup's natural ingredients. Although options (A), (C), and (D) describe qualities of the soup and how it should be prepared, they are not written in a persuasive manner and so are inappropriate for advertising a product.

A–19

(B) The manufacturer likely included nutritional information to keep consumers aware of what the soup contains. While people who want to work in food manufacturing or advertising might find interest in the presentation of the soup label, options (A) and (D) are incorrect because they are not likely the main reason for which nutritional information is listed on the label. Similarly, option (C) is incorrect because medical practitioners are not likely the main target audience of the nutritional information on the label.

Passage 3

Read the following passage and answer Questions 20 to 31.

Vitamin D

Vitamin D refers to a group of fat-soluble secosteroids, or steroids in which one of the bonds in the steroid rings is broken. When used without a subscript, the term "vitamin D" usually refers to vitamin D_2 and vitamin D_3.

Fat-soluble vitamins, such as vitamin D, are more likely to accumulate in the body than water-soluble vitamins, such as vitamin C, because they are absorbed through the intestinal tract with the help of lipids or fats. This means that vitamin D and other fat-soluble vitamins pose a greater risk for toxicity or hypervitaminosis because they are more difficult for the body to excrete.

Many vertebrates produce vitamin D in the skin after exposure to ultraviolet B light. Natural forms of the vitamin also can be found in a limited number of foods. Due to its perceived health and wellness benefits, vitamin D is commonly included in artificially fortified staple foods such as dairy and wheat products. It also can be found as a supplement in grocery and health-food stores.

Biological Processing

After it enters the body, vitamin D is sent to the liver. There, it is converted into calcidiol and then to calcitriol, which is the biologically active form of vitamin D. It is calcitriol that is known to protect the body. The synthesis of calcitriol in the kidneys causes it to circulate as a hormone, a process that controls the amount of calcium and phosphate in the bloodstream. This, in turn, strengthens the bones, which prevents osteoporosis, rickets in children, and a condition called hypocalcemic tetany, a neuromuscular disease caused by low levels of calcium in the bloodstream.

Vitamin D and Nutrition

Human beings produce vitamin D in the skin when they are exposed to the ultraviolet B rays from direct sunlight. However, many countries have fortified cereals, milk, margarine, yogurt, and bread products with vitamin D.

(Continued)

The U.S. Food and Nutrition Board recommends a daily allowance of 200 IU for children and adults under the age of 50, 400 IU for adults between 50 and 70, and 600 IU for adults over the age of 70. This daily intake amount represents an amount deemed sufficient to maintain bone health and the normal metabolism of calcium in healthy people. Despite the touted benefits of larger amounts of vitamin D by some researchers, intake of vitamin D above 2,000 IU a day is considered toxic by the U.S. Food and Nutrition Board.

Some people believe that vitamin D has the potential to prevent influenza, cancer, depression, and cardiovascular disease, though research in these areas shows mixed results.

Natural Sources of Vitamin D
The most common producers of natural vitamin D are fatty fish, such as salmon, catfish, and sardines. The only vegan source of vitamin D is found in mushrooms, after they have been exposed to sunlight.

Natural sources of vitamin D include:

Species	Serving Size	Amount of Vitamin D (IU)
Catfish	85 g (3 oz)	425
Salmon, cooked	100 g (3.5 oz)	360
Mackerel, cooked	100 g (3.5 oz)	345
Sardines, canned in oil, drained	50 g (1.75 oz)	250
Egg, whole	1 unit	20
Fish liver oils	1 tbsp (15 ml)	1,360

Questions

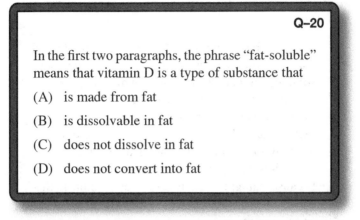

Q-20

In the first two paragraphs, the phrase "fat-soluble" means that vitamin D is a type of substance that

(A)   is made from fat

(B)   is dissolvable in fat

(C)   does not dissolve in fat

(D)   does not convert into fat

Your Answer _____

_____

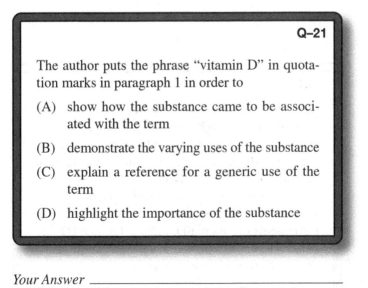

Q-21

The author puts the phrase "vitamin D" in quotation marks in paragraph 1 in order to

(A)   show how the substance came to be associated with the term

(B)   demonstrate the varying uses of the substance

(C)   explain a reference for a generic use of the term

(D)   highlight the importance of the substance

Your Answer _____

_____

Correct Answers

A–20

(B) The comparison between fat-soluble and water-soluble vitamins makes it clear that "fat-soluble" refers to the ease with which the vitamins are dissolvable in fat. While fat is involved in the processing of vitamin D, option (A) is incorrect because the passage states that vitamin D is a fat-soluble compound, rather than a type of fat itself. Similarly, options (C) and (D) are incorrect because paragraph 2 suggests that vitamin D dissolves in fat, which makes it more difficult to excrete from the body.

A–21

(C) The author puts the term "vitamin D" in quotes to highlight that the generic use of the term refers to vitamin D_2 and vitamin D_3. While the author discusses the molecular composition of vitamin D, option (A) is incorrect because there is no information included about how the vitamin got its name. Similarly, while the author discusses the benefits of vitamin D, options (B) and (D) are incorrect because the word is not put in quotes to discuss its uses or its importance.

Questions

Q–22

According to paragraph 2, "hypervitaminosis" is *most likely*

(A) a state of excess excretion

(B) a condition of vitamin overdose

(C) a state of insufficient vitamin intake

(D) a condition of nutritional equilibrium

Your Answer _____

_____

Q–23

For what reason does the author suggest that vitamin D is included in artificially fortified foods?

(A) It is a natural element in many foods.

(B) It is a required supplement to processed food.

(C) It is an important supplement to maintain health.

(D) It is a key element to keeping certain foods safe on the shelf.

Your Answer _____

_____

Correct Answers

A–22

(B) The passage states that hypervitaminosis is a type of toxicity, which suggests that it is a condition of "vitamin overdose." While the passage mentions the involvement of fat in the processing of vitamin D, option (A) is incorrect because it does not describe a condition of toxicity. Similarly, while the passage mentions the problems of insufficient levels of vitamin D, option (C) is incorrect because this is not a relevant description of the effects of toxicity. Finally, option (D) is incorrect because the passage makes it clear that hypervitaminosis is a case of toxicity rather than equilibrium.

A–23

(C) Vitamin D is critical to maintaining many key biological processes, such as the regulation of calcium and phosphate in the bloodstream. While some foods naturally contain vitamin D, option (A) is incorrect because vitamin D is added to foods in order to help people meet their daily requirements. Similarly, while there are regulations to the contents of processed food, option (B) is incorrect because the author does not provide any information about the required elements in processed food. Option (D) is incorrect because there is no suggestion that vitamin D is a preservative.

Questions

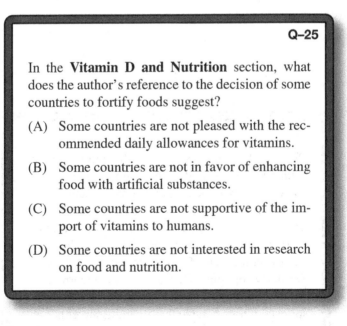

Q-24

According to the passage, what happens to calcitriol after it enters the kidneys?

(A) It is combined into a bioactive hormone.

(B) It is disintegrated into calcium and phosphate.

(C) It is separated into component hormone-like substances.

(D) It is absorbed by the bloodstream and re-enters the liver.

Your Answer _____

_____

Q-25

In the **Vitamin D and Nutrition** section, what does the author's reference to the decision of some countries to fortify foods suggest?

(A) Some countries are not pleased with the recommended daily allowances for vitamins.

(B) Some countries are not in favor of enhancing food with artificial substances.

(C) Some countries are not supportive of the import of vitamins to humans.

(D) Some countries are not interested in research on food and nutrition.

Your Answer _____

_____

Correct Answers

A–24

(A)   The author's use of the word "synthesis" suggests that calcitriol is transformed into a bioactive hormone when it enters the kidneys. While the biologically active form of vitamin D controls the regulation of calcium and phosphate in the bloodstream, option (B) is incorrect because there is no indication that calcitriol itself is transformed into these substances. Similarly, option (C) is incorrect because the author is discussing the synthesis or formation of calcitriol in the kidneys, not its separation. Also, option (D) is incorrect because there is no indication that calcitriol reverts and re-enters the liver after it is processed by the kidneys.

A–25

(B)   The author's use of the phrase "many countries" suggests that there are some countries that do not favor the artificial enhancement of food with vitamins. While it is possible that some countries do not favor the recommended allowances of vitamins, option (A) is incorrect because this is not a relevant inference for this section of the passage. Similarly, options (C) and (D) are incorrect because there is no indication from the passage that some countries believe that vitamins are either unimportant for research or for humans.

Questions

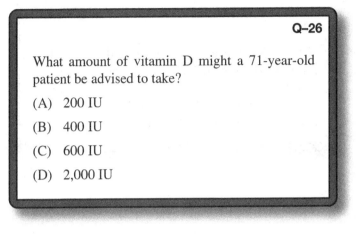

Q-26

What amount of vitamin D might a 71-year-old patient be advised to take?

(A) 200 IU

(B) 400 IU

(C) 600 IU

(D) 2,000 IU

Your Answer _____

_____

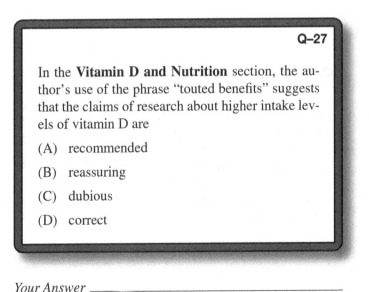

Q-27

In the **Vitamin D and Nutrition** section, the author's use of the phrase "touted benefits" suggests that the claims of research about higher intake levels of vitamin D are

(A) recommended

(B) reassuring

(C) dubious

(D) correct

Your Answer _____

_____

Correct Answers

A-26

(C) The passage states that 600 IU is the RDA for a person over the age of 70. Options (A), (B) and (D) are incorrect because these amounts are either significantly under or over the recommended daily amount for an adult over the age of 70.

A-27

(C) The phrase "touted benefits" suggests that the research claims are inconclusive or in doubt. While the author states that there are varying claims as to the effects of higher levels of vitamin D, options (A), (B), and (D) are incorrect because the author states that higher levels of vitamin D are deemed toxic by many researchers.

Questions

In the **Natural Sources of Vitamin D** section, the author suggests all of the following about vegans EXCEPT

(A) they may have to read food labels carefully to avoid non-animal forms of vitamin D

(B) they may have to rely upon supplements to meet their daily requirements of vitamin D

(C) they may have to eat mushrooms regularly to meet part of their daily vitamin D requirement

(D) they may have to start increasing their intake of fish in order to get enough vitamin D in their diets

Your Answer _____

_____

Correct Answers

A-28

(D) Vegans do not eat fish, so this would be an incorrect inference from this section and therefore the correct answer. Options (A), (B), and (C) are incorrect because they are all possible inferences from the author's statement that mushrooms are the only naturally available source of vitamin D for vegans.

Questions

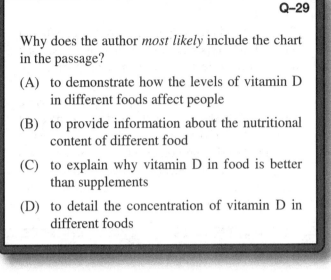

Q–29

Why does the author *most likely* include the chart in the passage?

(A) to demonstrate how the levels of vitamin D in different foods affect people

(B) to provide information about the nutritional content of different food

(C) to explain why vitamin D in food is better than supplements

(D) to detail the concentration of vitamin D in different foods

Your Answer _____

_____

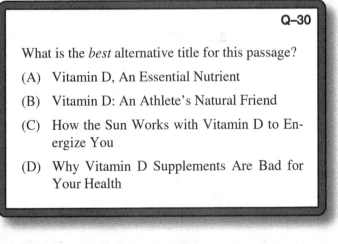

Q–30

What is the *best* alternative title for this passage?

(A) Vitamin D, An Essential Nutrient

(B) Vitamin D: An Athlete's Natural Friend

(C) How the Sun Works with Vitamin D to Energize You

(D) Why Vitamin D Supplements Are Bad for Your Health

Your Answer _____

_____

Correct Answers

A–29

(D) The chart explains the amount of vitamin D in different types of food. Although the passage discusses the effects of vitamin D on people, option (A) is incorrect because the chart does not detail how vitamin D affects people. Similarly, while the chart lists the vitamin D content of different foods, option (B) is incorrect because the chart does not describe any other nutrients. Finally, option (C) is incorrect because the chart does not explain why natural sources of vitamin D are better than supplements.

A–30

(A) The passage is a summary of vitamin D, how the body processes it, and its various health benefits. While the passage explains some of the positive benefits of vitamin D, option (B) is incorrect because the passage does not explain why it is good for athletes. Similarly, options (C) and (D) are incorrect because they discuss minor themes of the passage, rather than summarizing the passage itself.

Questions

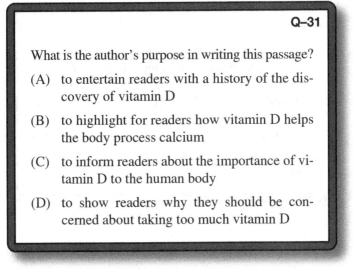

Q–31

What is the author's purpose in writing this passage?

(A) to entertain readers with a history of the discovery of vitamin D

(B) to highlight for readers how vitamin D helps the body process calcium

(C) to inform readers about the importance of vitamin D to the human body

(D) to show readers why they should be concerned about taking too much vitamin D

Your Answer _____

_____

Correct Answers

A–31

(C)   The passage is concerned with showing readers why vitamin D is important to the metabolism and function of the human body. Option (A) is incorrect because the author does not discuss the discovery of this nutrient. Similarly, options (B) and (D) are incorrect because they focus on minor details in the passage rather than a summary of the main idea.

Passage 4

Read the following passage and answer Questions 32 to 40.

Private Spaceflight

The private space industry is a growing part of the defense, communications, and transportation services market. Private spaceflight comprises orbital and sub-orbital flight over 100 km (62 mi) above Earth that is subsidized either by an individual or non-governmental entity.

In the 1950s and 1960s, the United States and other countries worked with private companies and other bodies to forge new space technologies at a rapid pace. These early collaborations led to the creation of the European Space Agency in 1975. By the mid-1970s, private companies and defense contractors began to invest seriously in space launch systems, realizing their revenue, communications, and intelligence-gathering potential.

Derived from governmental rockets, private spaceflight includes commercial communications satellites, satellite TV, satellite radio, and space tourism. While only major countries had funding to run space programs during the first few years of the space race, spaceflight evolved over time, particularly as technologies, defense system infrastructure, and funding sources improved. Eventually, regulations surrounding commercial space launches loosened, which paved the way for private organizations to offer and purchase space launches. For example, the U.S. Communications Satellite Act of 1962 paved the way for the first private spaceflights in the United States, involving the launch of early commercial communications satellites on government-owned launch vehicles.

In 1980, the European Space Agency initiated Arianespace to create the world's first commercial space transportation company. By 1997, Arianespace had made its one hundredth launch. The company has 23 shareholders, which include representatives from 10 different countries who work across a spectrum of scientific, financial, and political organizations. In 2003, Arianespace joined forces with several corporate partners to create the Launch Services Alliance in response to the evolving needs of the commercial and governmental markets.

(Continued)

In contrast to the public-private collaborations of the European space industry, private spaceflight has historically been much more restricted in the United States. Until the Commercial Launch Act of 1984, all commercial satellite launches had to be coordinated with NASA's space shuttle program. While commercial satellite launches on the space shuttle were initially subsidized, NASA initially had plans to introduce a commercial pricing system to maintain costs. Once the governmental monopoly on space launches ended, the number of commercial satellite launches increased dramatically. Ironically, the business of spaceflight changed so much by 1990 that even the U.S. government became a client. In November of 1990, President George W. Bush signed the Launch Services Act, which required the government to utilize commercial launch services for its regular activities when necessary.

In the last decade, the landscape for private spaceflight has changed dramatically. Private space transportation organizations now provide services for communications companies and government agencies around the world. The past few years also has seen growth in the space tourism industry, with companies like Virgin Galactic vying to provide space travel for private individuals. Additionally, astro-entrepreneurs have pioneered independent space systems to compete with government-sponsored space programs. These independent programs include ideas for sub-orbital spaceplanes, lightweight orbital rockets, solar sailing, personal moon spaceflights, and a private orbital living habitat.

Questions

Q–32

In the first paragraph, the author's use of the term "subsidized" suggests that

(A) governmental spaceflight costs less than non-governmental spaceflight

(B) governmental spaceflight is less regulated than other types of spaceflight

(C) non-governmental spaceflight receives financial support from commercial enterprise

(D) non-governmental spaceflight requires more commercial support than other businesses

---

Your Answer _____

_____

Correct Answers

A–32

(C) The word "subsidized" means "paid for" or "supported," which suggests that commercial enterprise provides financial support for non-governmental spaceflight. While the passage talks about the history of spaceflight regulation, options (A) and (B) are incorrect because the author does not mention the relative costs of private vs. government space programs. Similarly, while the author states that private spaceflight requires financial support from corporations and other entities, option (D) is incorrect because there is no suggestion that spaceflight is more expensive than other types of business.

Questions

Read the following paragraph.

Atmospheric flight is generally defined as flights under 100 km above sea level. On the other hand, sub-orbital and orbital flight comprises spaceflight over 100 km above sea level.

Based on the passage, what can be inferred from the above paragraph?

(A) 100 km above sea level is a dividing line between orbital flight and space.

(B) 100 km above sea level is a dividing line between sub-orbital and orbital flight.

(C) 100 km above sea level is a dividing line between Earth and its atmosphere.

(D) 100 km above sea level is a dividing line between Earth atmosphere and space.

Your Answer _____

_____

Correct Answers

A–33

(D) The passage states that sub-orbital and orbital flights are both categories of spaceflight. Building on this knowledge and the information about atmospheric flight in the given paragraph, it is clear that 100 km is the acknowledged dividing line between Earth's atmosphere and space. Option (A) is incorrect because orbital flight is a type of spaceflight, so this answer is redundant. Similarly, there is no information in either the passage or the paragraph to explain the difference between orbital and sub-orbital spaceflight, so option (B) is incorrect. While sea level is generally considered to be a dividing line between Earth and its atmosphere, option (C) is incorrect because 100 km is not a logical dividing point between Earth and its atmosphere.

Questions

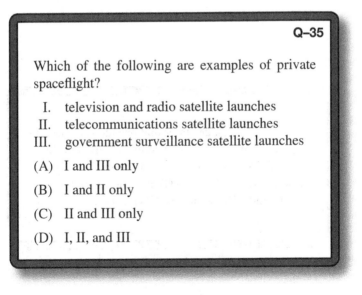

Q–34

In the 1970s, private organizations began investing in spaceflight technology because they believed that it would

(A) become a lucrative and important business

(B) give them an advantage over other organizations

(C) help governments cooperate better with each other

(D) enhance the pace of scientific development in other sectors

Your Answer _____

Q–35

Which of the following are examples of private spaceflight?

  I. television and radio satellite launches
 II. telecommunications satellite launches
III. government surveillance satellite launches

(A) I and III only

(B) I and II only

(C) II and III only

(D) I, II, and III

Your Answer _____

Correct Answers

A–34

(A) The passage makes it clear that private companies realized the future earning potential of the spaceflight industry. Options (B) and (D) are incorrect because there is no indication that companies interested in space technologies thought it would give them advantages over or assist business in other sectors. Similarly, there is no information to suggest that private companies thought that their investment in space technology would improve intergovernmental relations.

A–35

(B) The passage states that private spaceflights include "commercial communications satellites, satellite TV, satellite radio, and space tourism." Options (A), (C), and (D) are incorrect because they include III, which is NOT a type of private spaceflight.

Questions

In what order did the following events in early U.S. private spaceflight take place?

(A) NASA created, government purchases launch services from private sector, law about government launch of commercial satellites set up, restrictions on private spaceflight launches removed

(B) government purchases launch services from private sector, law about government launch of commercial satellites set up, restrictions on private spaceflight launches removed, NASA created

(C) laws about government launch of commercial satellites set up, NASA created, government purchases launch services from private sector, restrictions on private spaceflight launches removed

(D) NASA created, laws about government launch of commercial satellites set up, restrictions on private spaceflight launches removed, government purchases launch services from private sector

Your Answer _____

Correct Answers

A–36

(D) According to the passage, the United States first set up its governmental space agency, NASA, and then established laws restricting commercial satellite launches to the space shuttle but later removed these restrictions and found the need to purchase these private services. Options (A), (B), and (C) are incorrect because they do not correctly reflect the order of events described in the passage.

Questions

Q–37

Why does the author *most likely* include information about Arianespace in the passage?

(A) to contrast the European Space Agency's view toward private entities with that of the United States

(B) to compare the efficiency of European space-flight vehicles with those owned by the United States

(C) to compare the European Space Agency's funding sources with those of the United States

(D) to contrast the number of European space-flight launches with those of the United States

Your Answer _____

_____

Correct Answers

A–37

(A) The author likely includes information about the European space program to contrast its cooperation with private space organizations with the U.S. restrictions on these types of collaboration. While the author includes information about the number of Arianespace launches, option (B) is incorrect because there is no subsequent discussion of the efficacy of U.S. launch vehicles. Similarly, while the author suggests that Arianespace received funding from private sources, there is no comparison with the funding structures or number of launches of U.S. space vehicles, so options (C) and (D) are incorrect.

Questions

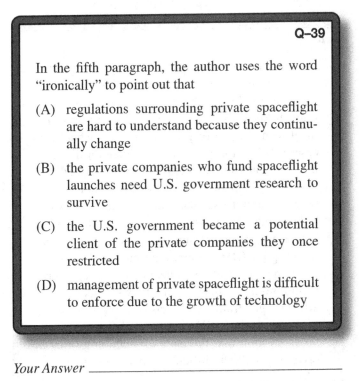

Q-38

As it is used in the fifth paragraph, the phrase "governmental monopoly" most nearly means

(A) governmental block

(B) governmental agency

(C) governmental control

(D) governmental research

Your Answer _____

Q-39

In the fifth paragraph, the author uses the word "ironically" to point out that

(A) regulations surrounding private spaceflight are hard to understand because they continually change

(B) the private companies who fund spaceflight launches need U.S. government research to survive

(C) the U.S. government became a potential client of the private companies they once restricted

(D) management of private spaceflight is difficult to enforce due to the growth of technology

Your Answer _____

Correct Answers

A–38

(C) The word "monopoly" means "control" or "domination," which refers to the U.S. government's full restrictions on commercial satellite launches to U.S. space shuttle flights. While the U.S. government did limit spaceflights to government launches, option (A) is incorrect because there were no blocks on these flights. Similarly, options (C) and (D) are incorrect because while a government agency was in charge of researching and implementing the programs that led to this type of legislation, these are not correct meanings of the word "monopoly."

A–39

(C) The author uses "ironically" to contrast the U.S. government's former restrictions on private spaceflight launches with the legislation of the Launch Services Act, which enables the government to make use of private launches when necessary. While the passage does mention different laws surrounding the regulation of spaceflight, option (A) is incorrect because it does not explain why the author uses the word "ironically." Similarly, while the passage discusses collaboration between government and private-sector organizations, option (B) is incorrect because there is no indication that private organizations require government funding to survive. Finally, while technology affected governmental decisions on spaceflight regulation, option (D) is incorrect because there is no suggestion that the pace of technology makes private spaceflight difficult to manage or regulate.

Questions

For whom is this passage *mainly* intended?

(A) people who are training to become astronauts

(B) people who enjoy reading about spaceflight pioneers

(C) people who want to invest in commercial space research

(D) people who are interested in the future of spaceflight programs

Your Answer _____

_____

Correct Answers

A-40

(D)   The author writes this passage for a general, nontechnical audience, which suggests that it would be most useful for people interested in the future of spaceflight programs. While potential astronauts and investors may want to read the history of spaceflight, they comprise only a part of the wider intended audience of this passage, so options (A) and (C) are incorrect. Similarly, option (B) is incorrect because there is no discussion of pioneers in spaceflight in the passage.

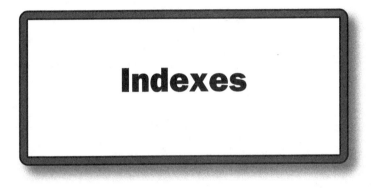

Indexes

Mathematics/Numerical Ability Index

Note: Numbers in the Index refer to question numbers.

Verbal Ability Index

Note: Numbers in the Index refer to question numbers.

Analogies, 8, 9, 32, 33,
56, 57, 80, 81, 103,
104

Antonyms, 6, 7, 30, 31,
54, 55, 78, 79, 101,
102

Capitalization, 16, 17,
40, 41, 64, 65, 88,
89, 111, 112

Language Use, 10, 11,
12, 13, 14, 15, 16,
17, 18, 19, 34, 35,
36, 37, 38, 39, 40,
41, 42, 43, 58, 59,
60, 61, 62, 63, 64,
65, 66, 67, 82, 83,
84, 85, 86, 87, 88,
89, 90, 91, 105, 106,
107, 108, 109, 110,
111, 112, 113, 114

Pronouns, 12, 13, 36, 37,
60, 61, 84, 85, 107,
108

Punctuation, 18, 19, 42,
43, 66, 67, 90, 91,
113, 114

Sentence Structure, 10,
11, 34, 35, 58, 59,
82, 83, 105, 106

Spelling, 20, 21, 22, 23,
24, 25, 44, 45, 46,
47, 48, 49, 68, 69,
70, 71, 72, 73, 92,
93, 94, 95, 96, 97,
115, 116, 117, 118,
119, 120

Subject-Verb
Agreement, 14, 15,
38, 39, 62, 63, 86,
87, 109, 110

Synonyms, 4, 5, 8, 29,
52, 53, 76, 77, 99,
100

Verbal ability, 1, 2, 3,
26, 27, 50, 51, 74,
75, 98

Science Ability Index

Note: Numbers in the Index refer to question numbers.

Science Ability Index

Note: Numbers in the Index refer to question numbers.

Reading Comprehension Index
Note: Numbers in the Index refer to question numbers.

Blank Cards for
Your Own Questions

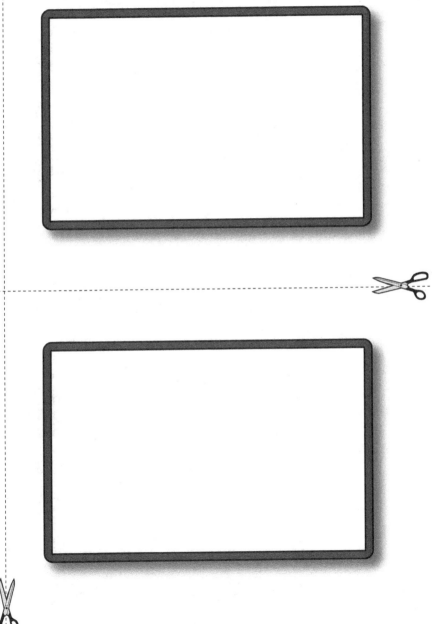

Correct Answers

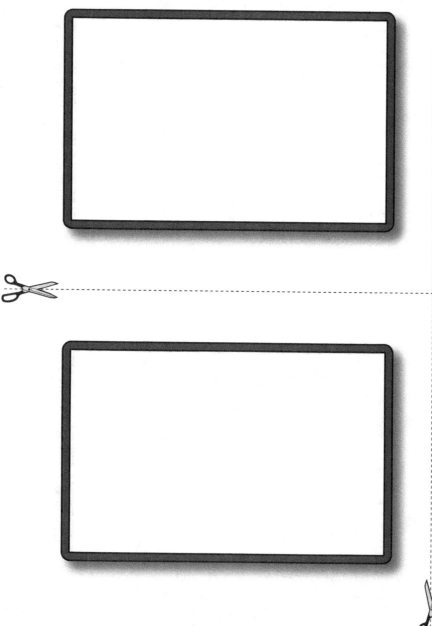

Blank Cards for
Your Own Questions

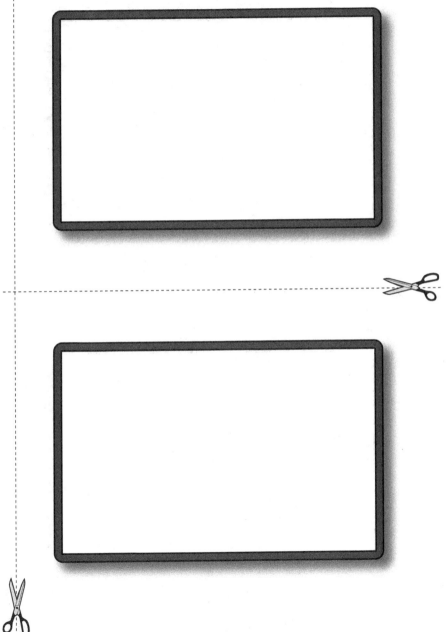

Correct Answers

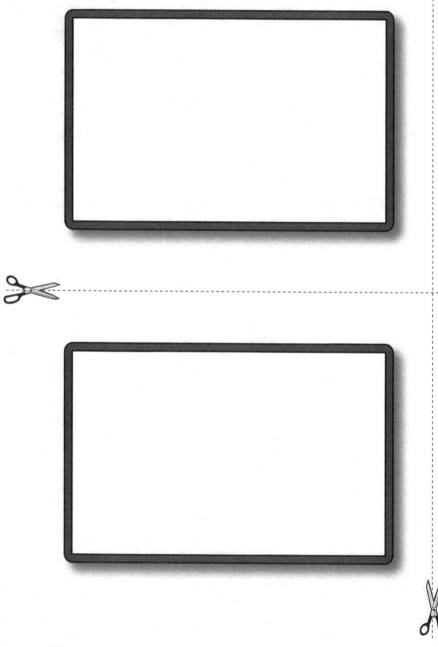

Blank Cards for Your Own Questions

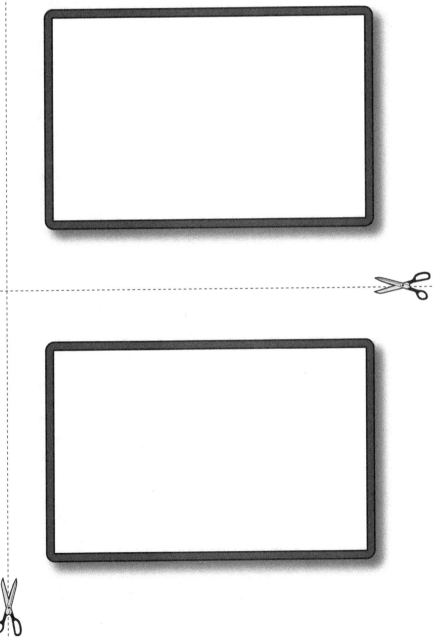

Correct Answers

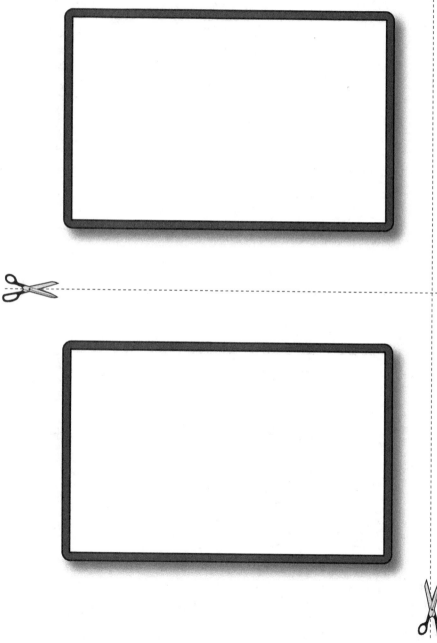

Blank Cards for
Your Own Questions

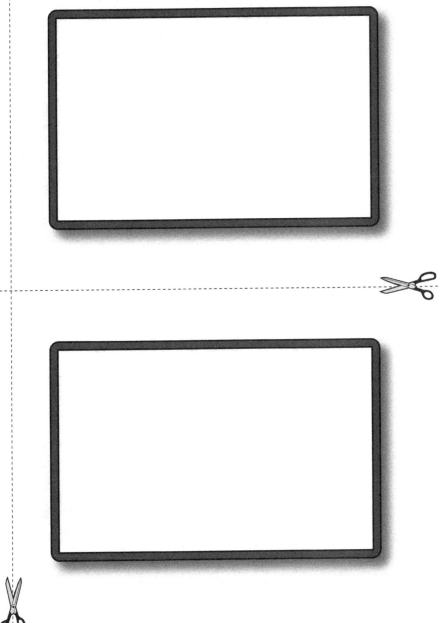

Correct Answers

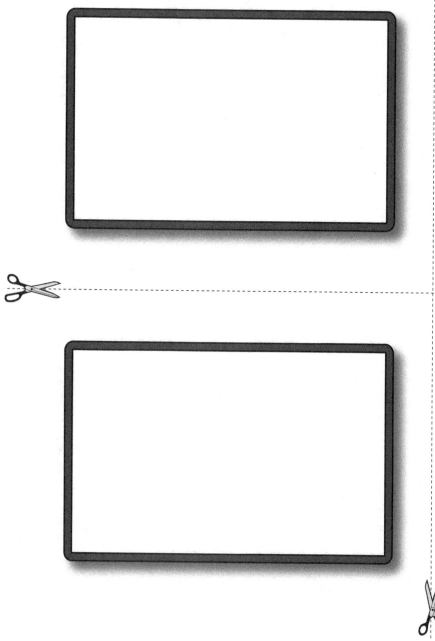

Blank Cards for
Your Own Questions

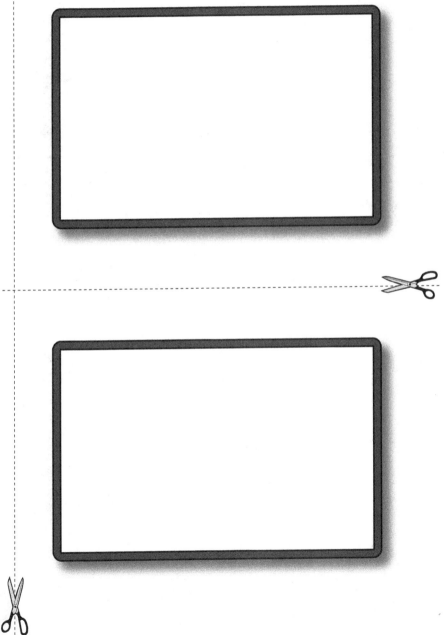

Correct Answers

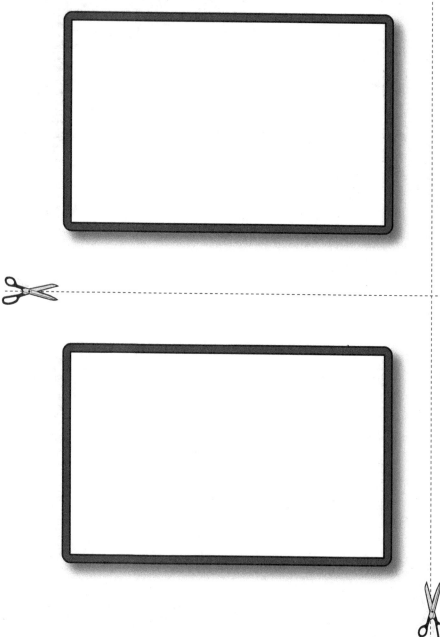

Blank Cards for
Your Own Questions

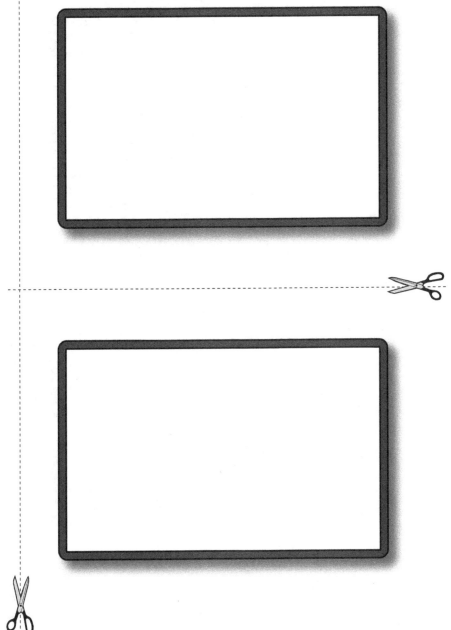

Correct Answers

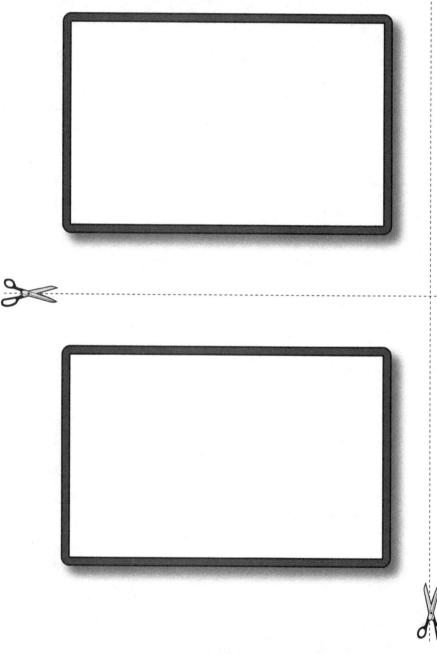